I0114815

FAITH

Fearlessly Affirming And Intending To Transform Health

Mylaine Riobé, MD, FABOIM, FACOG

Copyright © 2021 by Mylaine Riobé, MD, FABOIM, FACOG

All rights reserved. No part of this publication may be reproduced, distributed, or transmitted in any form or by any means, including photocopying, recording, or other electronic or mechanical methods without the prior written permission of the author, except in the case of brief quotations embodied in critical reviews and certain other non-commercial uses permitted by copyright law. For permission requests, write to the publisher:

Mylaine Riobé, MD
Riobé Institute of Integrative Medicine
Available on Amazon in print and kindle format

FAITH Fearlessly Affirming and Intending to Transform Health/Mylaine Riobé, MD, FABOIM, FACOG —1st ed.
ISBN 978-0-578-79127-2

I dedicate this book and its ideas to Truth: the unique path we all undertake in our lives to come to the shocking realization that we are much more than we're led to believe; the courage to stand in that Truth once it's found; and the strength to remain with it even when it's shaken.

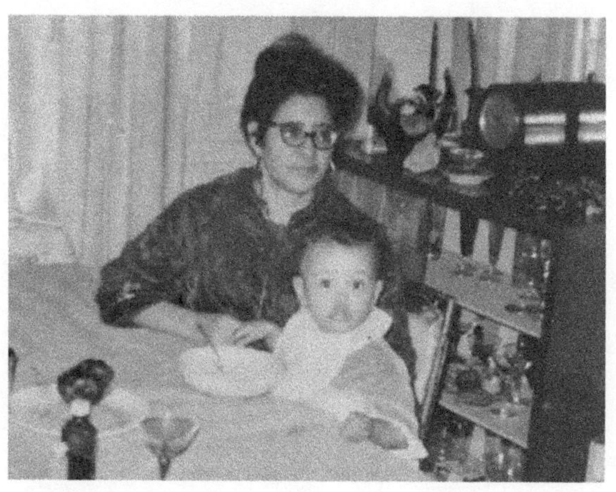

Mylaine with her grandma Armande Dougé, circa 1970

CONTENTS

INTRODUCTION

What is deep listening? We assume that we listen with our ears, but the great mystic poet Rumi asks us to reconsider what true listening is. In his poem "Listening" as translated by Coleman Barks, Rumi says:

"What is deep listening? Sama is a greeting from the secret ones inside the heart, a letter. The branches of your intelligence grow new leaves in the wind of this listening. The body reaches a peace."

"Give more of your life to this listening. As brightness is to time, so you are to the one who talks to the deep ear in your chest. I should sell my tongue and buy a thousand ears when that one steps near and begins to speak."

What is deep listening? Is it the hearing of noise or the listening for truth? Is hearing the same as listening? Rumi speaks of the secret ones inside the *heart.* He says that with deep listening, the branches of our intelligence grow new leaves. He then goes on to say that we should give more of our life to this listening.

When I wrote my first book, *The Tao of Integrative Medicine*, I set out to share what I had learned as a medical doctor for over 15 years that led me to take a radical new path in my career as an obstetrician-gynecologist and integrative/functional medical doctor, as well as in my own health and wellness. In addition to thousands of hours of study in medicine, I had been hearing spiritual teachers through books, courses, and one-on-one teaching, but I had not yet been listening deeply to the secret ones in my heart. While the facts in "The Tao" are accurate, something was missing. Since that time, I've learned to listen, deeply listen with my heart, and not my ears.

Listening is emotional – a distinctly feminine quality, which is often suppressed in Western societies. Although I'm a female, to make it in this world, I had to take on the very masculine qualities of competing, winning, staying on top, never backing down, and proving my point. And this served me well, but I came to the realization that overexpressing masculine qualities is what is creating chaos in our society and culture, including in our allopathic medical system. Men can be themselves in a masculine world, but women cannot always be themselves if they want to meet the criteria of success as we currently define it. Being deeply split between who we truly are and who we're trying to be in order to succeed, creates deep inner divisions that make us sick and unhappy. It's as though we're at war with ourselves – our Souls, the secret ones of which Rumi speaks, are whispering from our hearts for us to listen deeply for another path to fulfillment while our egos are screaming at us to keep hearing with our ears so we remain blind and deaf to Truth. We all eventually choose to find the Truth. Why? Because nothing else is real.

FAITH: ***F***earlessly ***A***ffirming and ***I***ntending to ***T***ransform ***H***ealth, is a conversation about Truth and it infuses what I've learned through deep listening that I hope will inspire you to choose your Truth and radically change how you view your health and wellness. Our personal health and wellness are the lynchpins of our lives. Without them, we're shadows of ourselves. **Our current health crisis or sickness crisis is a direct result of moving away from the lessons of nature and Truth**.

One of the biggest lessons I've learned throughout my life is that nature is, in fact, perfect. *It's simply our perception of nature that is imperfect.* Nature is a force or energy that is beyond human understanding. The more we try to figure it out, the more there is to figure out. It's endless and it's been here in the form of our Universe for at least 15 billion years doing just fine without human intervention. Nature is our biggest teacher if we choose to listen. Listen deeply.

When our perception of something is distorted, we think that the thing itself is imperfect, when it's our vision and hearing that are myopic and limited. As a medical student, I had a very limited view of the human body and how it worked because we studied it in a vacuum. We didn't look at how the body flows with its environment. We didn't look at the spirit and mind and how they interacted with the body. We didn't understand that the body, mind, and spirit are one. We mistakenly thought that nature was imperfect and caused problems in the body that we had to "fix."

We didn't appreciate that a lot of our ailments were of our own doing: the synthetic products we allowed into our environment, the stress we allowed into our lives, and the food choices we made. In our Western conventional allopathic medical model, it took us less than 200 years to practically run out of options to "fix" nature. Our antibiotics are becoming ineffective, we're running out of prescription drugs to fix the mess we've created, our life expectancy is declining for the first time in over 50 years, and some of the surgeries we performed are being shown to have long-term significant side effects. Our cancer therapies haven't worked either. In fact, they cause more cancer and sometimes life-long side effects. Despite spending more than any other country in the world on healthcare, 25 countries throughout the world have longer life expectancy than we do here in the U.S. while spending a fraction on their healthcare systems. The *New England Journal of Medicine* published an alarming study in 2005 predicting that for the first time in 200 years, a generation of children would not outlive its parents due to life-shortening childhood diseases!

Spending more money on the wrong priorities isn't a viable solution. We simply cannot outspend disease and we're learning this lesson the hard way as our children's life expectancies shorten and we're inundated with more and more diseases. Where did we go wrong? We've gone wrong in five ways:

1. We don't prevent diseases. We simply wait for them to take hold, then scramble to patch people up in order to prevent death.
2. We forget that nature is, in fact, perfect and have moved away from nature rather than learning from it.
3. We still don't understand that nature will not change itself to bend to our whims. Nature's universal laws are fixed and it's up to us to bend to it, not the other way around.
4. We haven't yet learned that when we flow with nature, we bring out the wholeness and perfection that already resides within us and it.
5. We haven't yet understood that technology cannot make us whole. A sick society is doomed to fail no matter how much technology it develops to try to prevent the inevitable.

One of the most significant discoveries in western medicine was the accidental discovery of penicillin by Dr. Alexander Fleming during World War 1. He later stated "I did not invent penicillin. Nature did that. I only discovered it by accident." Penicillin is a by-product of mold. The ancient Egyptians knew that this secretion of mold was antimicrobial and used it thousands of years ago.

The most profound lesson for us to learn is that nature does have the solution – often a better one than we can devise. Nature has built-in perfect balance. Just take a look at the night sky or at a flower blooming to appreciate this perfection and balance. Ancient energy-based systems of medicine such as TCM (traditional Chinese medicine) and Ayurveda developed in India, revere nature and consider it our biggest teacher. These systems of medicine have survived relatively unchanged for over 4,000 years. They flow with ancient traditions and philosophies such as Buddhism, Taoism, and Hinduism. Modern scientific inquiries are showing that many of these ancient principles and traditions are quite sophisticated and applicable today just as they were thousands of years ago. I'll discuss these discoveries throughout this book. The great teachers and physicians of these ancient philosophies and systems of medicine were apparently deeply in touch with nature and listened deeply to its guidance. As an integrative medical doctor, my biggest and most profound role in my patients' lives is to guide them back to the awareness of their perfection and wholeness.

In the West, we've isolated ourselves from these energy-based systems and nature itself to our own detriment and we've forgotten the truth of who and what we are. We've overutilized our western medical methods and allowed the pendulum to swing too far to one side. We've lost balance. A true health and wellness system guides you back to wholeness. To be healthy is to be healed. The definition of the word "doctor" is teacher or guide. A true healthcare system is one in which you are guided to **wholeness**...a wholeness that is already within you ready to be revealed and experienced.

Our allopathic system of medicine is life-saving in the case of acute life-threatening diseases like a heart attack or appendicitis. We have the best system of medicine in the world for these types of conditions. This same system consistently fails at both preventing diseases and successfully treating chronic conditions. This is where more natural, holistic energy-based systems of medicine can have a huge impact here in the West. Practicing an integrative style of medicine consisting of the use of western allopathic medicine only when needed, and natural, more holistic systems in all other circumstances, is the future of medicine and the key to recovering our wellness here in the West.

In this book, I hope to profoundly and permanently change the way you look at your health and wellness. It's clear that the human body is under assault to the point of being threatened with extinction. We're currently in a trial by fire for our own survival! My goal is to present a valid argument for a more balanced system that combines eastern, natural energy-based forms of medicine with our western allopathic model that allows the pendulum to swing back to center so we can regain our wellness and reverse this disturbing trend towards self-destruction.

To help you build on what you'll learn here and implement these strategies in your life and career, **Awakened Wellness Nation** is our private online community where you'll find like-minded people ready to share their stories, insights and experiences. The principles of natural, holistic energy-based systems of medicine are simple and profound, but so different than our western thinking, that they're very challenging for us to comprehend. It's simply not part of our cultural conversation. What I've learned is priceless and I look forward to sharing these ideas with you in a way that you can incorporate so we can begin to have a different conversation about wellness here in the west. Whether you're a layperson looking to improve your health or a medical professional looking for a better way, this book and online community will help you forge that path.

The Truth is simple and profound: **we are a creation of nature and are one with it**. When we listen deeply with our hearts and look within, we can hear and see it. Some call it intuition, some call it Soul, and others call it God. Whatever it's called, it sits unchanged, eternal and whispering to us to seek Truth. I hope to inspire you to have

FAITH: ***F***earless ***A***ffirmation and ***I***ntention to ***T***ransform ***H***ealth. Choose to love yourself first each and every day to bring your best self to the world where we need you the most! Namaste.

HOW TO USE THIS BOOK

This book is for both lay people who wish to begin to understand why they can't get satisfactory answers from their physicians, and for healthcare professionals who feel that something is wrong with our current paradigm and are looking for a better way. Once we follow the facts, the cracks in our system become obvious and alarming; but the good news is that the facts also take us to a better place.

The style of medicine accepted as the standard of care here in the U.S. is called allopathic medicine. When medical students graduate and are awarded a doctorate of medicine or MD degree, it's in allopathic medicine. Other words used to describe it are Western medicine or conventional medicine.

Integrative medicine is a very broad term used to define any system of medicine that integrates with our allopathic model. Functional medicine is a modern holistic system of medicine that can be integrated with our allopathic system. The term integrative medicine should not be confused with internal medicine. *Internal* medicine developed in the 1800s as "evidence-based" medicine to be applied to the diagnosis and treatment of diseases commonly affecting adults. *Integrative* medicine is distinctly different in its practice and paradigm. Being holistic, it focuses on wellness, prevention and the physician-patient relationship. It incorporates mind, body and spirit in its practice.

Traditional Chinese medicine (TCM) is an ancient energy-based holistic system of medicine that originated in China about 4,000 years ago. It's still practiced there and in many countries throughout the world to this day. Acupuncture and Chinese herbal medicinals are used in TCM. I'll refer to traditional Chinese medicine as TCM throughout this book. It, too, can be integrated with our allopathic system. When TCM physicians speak of organs, they're not referring only to physical structures, but to energy fields that have certain functions within and beyond the body. As we'll see throughout this book, modern science is showing us that essentially everything is energy. We can detect this energy using various technologies as we'll see. To distinguish TCM organs from the physical structures that we recognize as organs in allopathic medicine, I've underlined the TCM organs.

In my private medical practice, I fuse traditional Chinese medicine with functional medicine and allopathic medicine. I reserve our allopathic system for acute, potentially life-threatening situations and use TCM and functional medicine for preventive strategies and to find and resolve root causes of symptoms and conditions when they're not life-threatening.

In order to improve retention of these points and ideas, I take a deeper dive into these principles in *The Wellness Warrior 9-Week Transformation Program*. To get the most out of a new concept, it's important to have repetition, reinforcement, and examples so you can apply them to your everyday life. This is why I decided to add online courses for my clients. My clients have greatly benefited from a disruptive approach to their health – concepts that are radical, effective, natural, and based in science. I've also benefited from an approach that helps me guide clients to better health. I reference medical studies as well as ancient texts throughout this book to reinforce ideas. My ideas are not new. They can be found in ancient texts that are thousands of years old as well as in cutting-edge modern research. This research is often not found in mainstream medical journals commonly read by allopathic physicians and go unnoticed by the medical community in the West.

What will motivate change will be consumer demand for a better, more effective way to maintain wellness and healthcare practitioners who believe in a better way to forge the path. I hope that this book, our online community and programs will inspire such demand and change.

CHAPTER ONE

WHERE ARE WE?

Home Is Where The Heart Is

Growing up in a Caribbean family in NYC helped shape my mind in ways I'll probably never fully comprehend. I owe my open-mind to the Big Apple! Although I currently reside in Florida, NYC will always be my home.

I loved learning about the different people, beliefs and cultures that surrounded me there. I could see that they all had a similar end in mind, and a seemingly infinite number of ways to get there! They all seemed so different, yet the same. I didn't understand what the "sameness" about them was at the time, but sensed it nonetheless. They all had a certain faith, but chose to express it differently. When we examine this faith at its core, it's really the same for all philosophies. All major philosophies advise us to go within to seek the Truth: from Buddhism to Hinduism, to Christianity, to Judaism… so why all the discord and strife? I call this iceberg syndrome. We stay on the surface and ignore what's underneath. We focus on semantics rather than the core message. When we finally look beyond the semantics, we realize that the differences are so miniscule as to be ignored.

Our current health crisis is very similar. We focus so intently on what's on the surface that we've forgotten to look beneath the surface to go within to find the source or root cause of the problem. This iceberg syndrome approach has led us astray with tunnel vision that has now reached disastrous proportions. The *New England Journal of Medicine* published a study in 2005, predicting that our children born of this generation are projected to have shorter lifespans than we do for the first time in 200 years! In fact, we've already begun to see this unfathomable statistic coming to fruition. The life expectancy in the U.S. has officially declined for the past 2 out of 3 years according to the Centers for Disease Control.

50% of American children are projected to have at least one chronic disease before the age of 18 according to a study published in June 2011 by the Journal *American Pediatrics*. All this technology and information, yet we seem to be going backwards, not forwards. What's going on? Some would have you believe that we should expect diseases because of all the great advancements that have contributed to us living longer. We're told that the reason we don't feel well and have diseases is because we're getting older and living longer. This statistic published by the *New England Journal of Medicine* regarding the shortened life expectancy of our children is a sobering wakeup call that this idea that we get sick because we live longer is simply untrue.

What's really going on? When the foundation of a system is flawed, all that comes from that broken foundation is equally flawed. When a system of medicine endeavors to look for diseases to treat using artificial and superficial means rather than preventing them and maintaining wellness, it keeps finding diseases after they've taken hold and soon becomes overwhelmed with more and more diseases. We've seen an explosion of new diseases in the past 100 years: allergic rhinitis, autoimmune disorders, asthma, autism, and attention deficit disorder, just to name a few. And many of these diseases are plaguing our children, making the argument that we're getting sicker because we're living longer a lot harder to believe.

Even diseases like cancer that have been around for thousands of years have seen an explosion of new cases. The latest estimates show that 42% of Americans will have a diagnosis of cancer by the year 2025. Cancer will soon surpass heart attacks as the number one killer of Americans.

As we've focused on finding "cures" for cancers using artificial means such as chemotherapy, radiation, and now, immunotherapy, we've paved the way for new types of cancers to take hold. While death from certain cancers such as cervical and breast cancer is improving, other cancers such as human papilloma virus-associated oropharyngeal cancer (a type of throat cancer), esophageal adenocarcinoma, pancreatic, liver, thyroid, and kidney cancers are on the rise! Why? Because we're paving the way for cancer when we're not focused on preventing it or maintaining a state of wellness.

Our current allopathic healthcare approach is akin to the game of "whack-a-mole," but this is hardly a game when lives are at stake. *The focus of allopathic medicine is to prevent DEATH from disease rather than to prevent the disease itself.* While that model works for acute life-threatening diseases like a heart attack or appendicitis, it doesn't work for the vast majority of health problems we face today. Our allopathic model excels at saving lives in the case of immediately life-threatening conditions like a heart attack or appendicitis, and has lost its focus on disease *prevention* and wellness. Instead, it waits for diseases, chases them, and treats them with superficial and often artificial means, which has been its downfall and the main reason that we're currently losing the battle to regain our health. Our vision has become astoundingly myopic.

When your life is in immediate danger, it's acceptable to save your life by any means necessary including using artificial and synthetic means, *but it becomes dangerous when this strategy is employed across the board for all conditions and symptoms, both chronic and acute.*

Allopathic medicine is hardly alone in the use of superficial and artificial means. We find this problem everywhere. Our household products such as cleaners, lotions, pesticides, plastics, genetically modified foods, pollution from industrial factories, and even some vitamins, are made of artificial ingredients and wreak havoc on the body's systems. Our body isn't prepared to deal with the constant exposure to synthetic and artificial products that it endures today.

The long-term use of artificial products in allopathic medicine and the constant exposure to artificial products in our homes and workplace have led us directly to our current health crisis. Our health crisis has also led to a fragile economy. While latest reports claim that our economy is holding its own, it's clear that Americans cannot hold onto their wealth as they age. Why? *We cannot outspend disease no matter how much money we have*. Our health IS our wealth. Health and wealth are inextricably connected in every way. Without an emphasis on wellness and prevention, we'll continue to spiral down into an unsustainable existence.

Our focus and foundation must change to prevention of disease using natural methods ***and a focus on wellness***. Prevention and wellness are very different, and a distinction should be made. Science is showing us clearly that our thoughts and focus create our reality and experiences. The focus on preventing a disease still brings the idea of disease itself into our awareness which increases its likelihood to take hold; whereas a focus on wellness excludes disease from our awareness, which makes it less likely to take hold. That's an important distinction to make when considering a wellness approach. I purposely de-emphasize disease with my private clients in order to reduce the focus on disease and increase the focus on wellness. This doesn't mean that we ignore diseases. It means that we don't give them a stronghold in our subconscious minds, which is where we create our perceptions and realities. I'll discuss this idea throughout this book because it's the pillar of wellness and wholeness. We literally become what we think.

What's the long-term solution? A true solution is to apply allopathic medicine only in the cases of immediately life-threatening diseases while applying more effective, already-existing preventive systems of medicine such as functional medicine and traditional Chinese medicine (collectively known as integrative medicine) over time to reduce the current disease burden that plagues our nation and increasingly, the world. Trying to twist our current American allopathic system of medicine into a "preventive" system when that isn't, and will likely never be its focus, will keep this solution from coming to fruition. We must apply already-established systems of medicine whose primary focus is wellness in order to begin to move in a better direction and reserve our allopathic system for immediately life-threatening diseases like heart attacks and appendicitis.

The first step is to admit we have a problem. ***Our American allopathic healthcare model is failing***, not because it's too expensive, not because of insurance companies and government regulations, but *simply because* ***its very foundation is ill-conceived***. We cannot focus on preventing death from disease because that plan is doomed to fail. We MUST focus on prevention of disease itself and shift to a "maintenance of wellness" model which already exists in other systems of medicine. We have to begin to look underneath the surface using systems of medicine that are better equipped than our own - systems that have a foundation of wellness - to climb out of this crisis and find our health and wellness once again.

This takes FAITH: **F**earlessly **A**ffirming and **I**ntending to **T**ransform **H**ealth! I'll discuss with you two systems of medicine that, when combined with allopathic medicine, give us the ability to more successfully promote wellness and treat existing diseases from a firm and sound foundation rather than one that is fundamentally flawed. I'll share these integrative principles to help you change your mindset to one of wellness rather than drinking the Kool-Aid® that says we just have to wait like sitting ducks for diseases to treat.

The *active promotion* of wellness is paramount and consists of more than just getting physical exams, blood work, mammograms, and colonoscopies at the appropriate timeframes. We call the physical exam, screening tests, and blood work obtained in our American allopathic model a preventive exam. This notion is fundamentally flawed. There's nothing preventive or wellness-promoting about getting a physical exam, blood work and a mammogram. A mammogram is designed to find abnormal breast densities on x-ray that may be cancer. Then a surgeon performs a biopsy of these areas of suspicion to either diagnose or rule out cancer. ***This isn't prevention. This is early diagnosis of disease***...and it's not even that early. The average breast cancer diagnosis is 7 years in the making! Prevention and wellness by definition are the absence of disease, not its early diagnosis.

So, the answer to the original question posed at the beginning of this chapter: "Where are we?" The simple answer is we're lost! How did we go so wrong in our allopathic medical system? *Our allopathic system is a mirror of our flawed thinking in our modern western society*. We seem to be trapped in the superficial and afraid to look deeply into ourselves. We prefer what we falsely believe is a quick fix to the work of prevention largely because prevention isn't even part of our cultural jargon here in the west.

We launch new technology such as the internet, then wait for all hell to break loose from the lack of planning, then scramble to fix the mess. We wait for bridges to collapse then pay out the lawsuits and move on rather than examining the infrastructure for weaknesses and flaws to correct. We move forward in the name of so-called progress even when we know that the potential consequences will be dire. While this approach seems immediately counterproductive, we see countless examples of this illogical thinking. Why? Because of the brain's survival mechanisms, we prefer to be comfortable in the known rather than risk the discomfort of looking more deeply into the unknown even when the known outcome is potentially catastrophic. The most alarming and poignant example of this is addiction. Although we intuitively know that the substances we're abusing such as alcohol, cigarettes or narcotics are dangerous and life-threatening, our brains trigger behavior that results in the immediate gratification of a perceived need for the drug despite the tremendous danger of this continued behavior. We know very clearly that cigarettes kill, narcotics kill, and excess alcohol kills, yet when addicted, we continue to exhibit this life-threatening behavior because *our brains are wired to function in this way*. For behaviors that are not as immediately life-threatening, our brains can work against us in many ways and we don't always make these connections because *we've been socialized to think from a fear-based perspective.* So, although we know that smoking cigarettes is life-threatening, we do it anyway because it immediately relieves stress. There are some evolutionary advantages to this type of brain function that we've now outgrown but continue to exhibit.

One of the many functions of our brain is to identify risks to our immediate survival - a critical function. Our brains which house our ego-based thoughts, are critical fight-or-flight organs. They're one of the main reasons our species was able to survive in its environment hundreds of thousands of years ago. Our brains are expert at detecting rapid motion, threatening sounds, and other dangers so we can mount a defense. But when this fight-or-flight response is carried to an extreme and remains unchecked, this survival instinct backfires, leading to the framing of our experiences from a place of fear. Fear-based thinking tends to promote behavior that will be immediately rewarding regardless of long-term consequences. It's like comfort food! It's yummy now but we'll pay later. It's irrational, yet comfortable in the moment because it allows us to retreat from having to fix the problem…so we think.

We prefer a drug that masks a symptom so we don't have to experience it, only to have it haunt us later with an even more difficult situation. The *fear* of the pain leads to the use of the drug to mask the pain. The pain itself isn't the motivator, it's our *fear* of pain that's the primary motivator.

During my 20 years of professional experience, I've come to realize that there are two categories of people who experience illness:

1. Those who see their illness as a means of learning and growth to more fully participate in their lives. These people are able to transcend the ego-based, fear-based thinking patterns that contribute to their diseases.
2. Those who see illness as a means of retreating from their lives. These people have not yet outgrown the ego-based, fear-based thinking patterns that contribute to their diseases.

The difference between these two groups is subtle, but profound. It all boils down to fear – the fear of life itself and the fear of the Truth that is buried deep within. Those who fearlessly affirm and intend to transform their health do, and those who remain in fear, may subconsciously sabotage themselves and remain sick. Fear is a powerful motivator and loosening the mind from its grip takes conscious, persistent practice and nurturing – especially when the fear is subconscious and we're not even aware that it exists. Whether you're in the first or second category, this book is for you!

I've found that far fewer people are in the first category than the second. I believe, based on the principle that we become what we think, that because the majority of people exhibit fear-based thinking, this momentum allowed our "sickness" care system to take hold over the past couple centuries. But in our new awareness, we're realizing that subconscious fears are holding us back from expressing our highest selves and many of us are seeking and finding a better way.

Because wellness and prevention are not a significant part of our cultural jargon, they're not part of the doctor's visit either. The annual so-called preventive exam is the primary example. We perform a physical exam, obtain blood work, pap smears for women at the appropriate timeframe, colonoscopy when indicated, and other testing. The idea of stress management, exercise and nutrition rarely, if ever, enter the conversation despite being critical to true prevention and management of disease. How did this happen? It starts at the foundation: medical education.

I attended Columbia University for my undergraduate pre-medicine studies and later New York Medical College, both very intellectual, dogmatic and competitive environments. Still in the heart of N.Y.C., I remained immersed in different cultures and religious philosophies. I kept looking for common threads among them to reconcile the differences. I noticed that as people got older, they allowed their differences to divide them rather than unite them. I'd later come to realize that this was rooted in fear-based thinking! I felt that finding common ground in philosophies would somehow help me in the future. Over the course of the next twenty years, I realized that finding common ground with an open mind helps you integrate theories and philosophies to better understand and embody them. It allows you to use the best of all the systems and discard what doesn't serve the highest good. While we learn a lot in medical school, being open-minded isn't one of the lessons, but my early years in N.Y.C. kept my mind open enough to keep looking and learning. I'm sharing what I've learned with you in this book in the hopes of forever changing how you think about your health and wellness.

The pursuit of a degree in allopathic medicine is extremely challenging and competitive. The average medical school applicant applies to about 15 schools and has between a 50-75% chance of being rejected from every single one of them! Can you say "fear-based thinking?" And the competition doesn't end there because following medical school admission, there's the rigorous and competitive curriculum which instills fear. The subjects are complex and difficult, and in order to get into a competitive residency program afterwards, you have to stay on top of your game. At no point in time do you get to relax. That's approximately 12-15 years of biting, scratching and clawing your way to your career path. And if you're not introspective in order to maintain work-life balance, you can easily go astray, which is what I believe has happened to the health industry in general and many other professions and industries. The imbalance inherent in a medical education and the profession itself is made even more blatant by the statistics that doctors have the highest rate of suicide and drug use of any profession. Medical doctors have twice the suicide rate as the general population. Something has to change.

Aside from the fear-based thinking instilled in the pursuit of a medical degree and the practice itself, there's also the deductive nature of the industry. Allopathic medicine is largely anatomical and physical; we deductively examine and investigate organs and how they form systems. In other words, we divide things into smaller components to understand them better but *we never look at how they influence each other and work together as a whole*. In medical school, we dissected cadavers and looked under microscopes to see what was "inside," so to speak. These procedures were necessary and important in order to learn to diagnose diseases and successfully treat them, but we *lost the holistic view of wellness and health in favor of hunting disease.* Even more astonishingly, we neglected the individual who had the disease in the first place, focusing solely on the disease and not the person.

I learned to diagnose and treat diseases, which is the paradigm of medical training in residency. This method seemed rather cookie-cutter considering the topics I had to master to get to that point. Every patient with a certain diagnosis received the same medical treatment. I didn't realize then that this wasn't a great way to practice medicine because it was all I was taught during residency. Nonetheless, I expected to be able to help countless people upon graduation, but rapidly became frustrated because I couldn't help my patients as I originally thought. Many of my clients suffered from fatigue, poor sleep, weight gain, sexual dysfunction, depression and anxiety, and I really couldn't help them. There wasn't a "disease" to treat in these cases. I tried. I prescribed medications as per my training — antidepressants, birth control pills, sleeping pills — but they didn't seem to work. Some felt better, but many returned with the same complaints and sometimes side effects.

In residency we were trained to look for diseases and, when absent, tell patients everything was normal. If they persisted in their complaints, we suggested that it was all in their heads or that they were depressed or maybe getting old. Ultimately, however, I was faced with a daunting reality. These symptoms weren't part of a disease complex, per se, they were just a series of random symptoms that I couldn't fix despite 13 years of advanced medical training. These symptoms appeared random until I further explored the field of traditional Chinese medicine and learned that there's **no such thing as random**!

Traditional Chinese medicine (TCM) resonated well because it flowed with my personal philosophy: one that blended Taoist and Buddhist philosophies with Christian principles because I found a lot of common threads between the three that were well expressed in TCM. TCM is a holistic energy-based system of medicine. Energy-based essentially means that it doesn't utilize what we could consider to be physical organs and anatomical structures. For example, the acupuncture points used in TCM are not anatomically visible like blood vessels or nerves, but they can be located using devices that detect electricity called impedance meters, although the "wires" through which the electricity or energy flows cannot be seen. Just as we can't see the electricity that flows through the wires that power our devices, we can't see acupuncture points and meridians; but just like electricity, the acupuncture points and meridians are definitely there.

Studying traditional Chinese medicine was far more difficult than I anticipated. My brain was so hard-wired for the deductive physical methods to diagnose and treat diseases that the more holistic energy-based philosophy that flowed through traditional Chinese medicine was extremely difficult for me to grasp despite how it correlated with my personal philosophies. So, I took an unconventional path in my pursuit.

As a medical doctor in this country, I'm granted a lot of freedom to incorporate different procedures and techniques into my practice. While I could have taken a short acupuncture course and incorporated it, I was quite fortunate to recognize that Chinese medicine was much more complex and profound than we're led to believe in the West and worthy of deeper study. There was much to learn to properly incorporate TCM into my practice, so I studied it for five years instead of the required 6 months. I completed a total of over 1000 hours of course work instead of the required 100 hours of course work. I completed a voluntary two-year internship with my mentors, Liping

Chang, M.D., LAc, and Fu Di, M.D., LAc. In China, Doctors of Oriental Medicine or acupuncturists are usually medical doctors who acquire a profound medical background with which to practice TCM. Here in the U.S. our standards for TCM education are more relaxed and that's made it difficult for us to truly appreciate the power of this comprehensive energy-based system of medicine. As I'll explain throughout this book, the new buzzword in health and indeed all of existence is ENERGY, and incorporating energy-based systems into our culture will be a turning point in our society. The famous inventor Nikola Tesla said of energy, "The day science begins to study non-physical phenomena, it will make more progress in one decade than in all the previous centuries of its existence."

Thanks to my studies and my mentors, I began to truly understand traditional Chinese medicine. With their blessing and encouragement, I incorporated TCM into my practice and never looked back. Symptoms that seemed random in allopathic medicine were very specifically related and fell nicely into patterns identified in Chinese medicine. Later in this book, I'll explain the theories of TCM that explain symptoms much more comprehensively than our allopathic model. My mentor in TCM, Dr. Fu Di, taught me a profound lesson that I continue to carry with me throughout my career. In TCM, Chinese herbal formulas are used to treat various patterns of disharmony that are assessed to be causing certain symptoms. Chinese herbal formulas consist of multiple single herbs blended together to treat the ***root cause*** of a symptom or pattern. Usually one formula is used and customized with the addition or subtraction of herbs to achieve the best match for each individual patient. Dr. Fu Di practices Chinese medicine in a most unconventional way, blending several different formulas and homeopathic remedies together to treat his patients because he says that Americans are different and have more complex health conditions than the Chinese. As Americans, we're overmedicated, acutely stressed, and just different than the Chinese so the methods that work in China won't necessarily work here in the United States. Knowing this, Dr. Fu Di incorporated his unconventional method into his practice with wonderful results. This had a profound impact on my practice of medicine. We are different. Things that worked for the Chinese didn't work quite as well for us. While my results after incorporating TCM were wonderful, I noticed a few conditions weren't as successfully treated with these methods. I knew I needed to look further for answers.

Enter Functional Medicine

Although functional medicine is also holistic, focusing on mind and body as a whole, it's also physical, anatomical, and deductive, just like our allopathic mainstream medicine. Chinese medicine (TCM), also a holistic system, is an energy-based system of medicine. Unlike allopathic medicine or even functional medicine, TCM exhibits little anatomical or deductive qualities, yet it works extremely well. I studied functional medicine to complement TCM. Functional medicine relies heavily on methods of testing that are drastically different than our allopathic system, so I learned to perform and interpret a lot of functional tests which specifically look inside of our body's cells and directly at our metabolism and energy production and utilization. I'll illustrate in chapter 9 why using blood work steers us in the wrong direction and how the use of cellular-based and metabolic testing is more appropriate for today's health needs. Incorporating TCM and functional medicine allowed me to look at symptoms and conditions from three different perspectives or angles, which provide a unique view of an individual's overall physical and mental condition.

I learned to use bio-identical hormone therapy, a natural form of hormone therapy. This was a big help because right after I obtained my board certification in OB/GYN in 2004, a study was published titled "The Women's Health Initiative Study" that contained devastating news for hormone replacement therapy in the United States. Synthetic- and pharmaceutical-grade hormones used to treat menopause symptoms in the U.S. for over 40 years were found to cause an increased risk of breast cancer and stroke after five years of use. This created a huge challenge because hormone replacement therapy is a cornerstone of gynecology, so I lost a big tool. Discovering bio-identical hormone replacement therapy helped me retool! I was free to treat menopausal symptoms if Chinese medicine wasn't helping me successfully treat these often-severe symptoms. So began my journey to blend all three very different medical systems into my practice, and the results have been terrific! In my quest for answers, I learned a valuable lesson: *I achieve better results when I blend systems together and use the best parts of each of them, rather than confine my treatment to one system.*

Using multiple systems of medicine works well because people are very unique and dynamic. We're never the same twice and we're unlike any other human being on the planet. We're not the same today as we were yesterday, and we won't be the same tomorrow as we are today. We are incessantly changing. Therefore, we need a dynamic system of medicine or blending of different systems of medicine that will keep up with those every-day changes and allow those changes to occur in a more harmonious and natural way. TCM and functional medicine help us to see beneath the surface to find root causes or risk factors not visible with our allopathic medical system. In other words, these holistic health systems look for and correct the weaknesses in the infrastructure before the bridge collapses!

In my private practice, I specifically use TCM to start all my evaluations to determine the underlying root causes of chronic conditions and symptoms which are called patterns of disharmony. Specific patterns of disharmony have specific food, herb, acupuncture, and lifestyle prescriptions to help balance the disharmony. I prescribe customized nutrition and lifestyle plans, herbal formulas, and acupuncture for these patterns of disharmony to restore balance and treat the underlying root causes.

I also use the patterns of disharmony to guide specific testing according to functional medicine principles, rather than chasing symptoms in an effort to find their causes. I already know the causes energetically, so I can drill into these causes with testing to complement that knowledge instead of stabbing in the dark as we often do in allopathic and functional medicine. After several years of practicing in this integrative-holistic way, I realized that I was not diagnosing people with diseases at the same rate that I had been when I was practicing allopathic medicine. My clients were healthier overall and felt much better. Yes, some still develop diseases due to factors beyond their control, but overall, they're much healthier than they otherwise would've been.

My results proved to me that the studies conducted in Europe and throughout the world on the effectiveness of Chinese and functional medicine were valid. In 2014, the American Board of Medical Specialties formally accepted the field of Integrative Medicine as a medical specialty. This legitimized what was once considered a fringe system of medicine. I obtained my board certification in August of 2017 to complement my board certification in OB-GYN.

Integrative medicine is the blending of different modalities with allopathic mainstream medicine. In my private practice, integrative medicine is specifically the blending of traditional Chinese medicine, functional medicine, allopathic medicine, and spiritual principles.

Integrative medicine helps prevent diseases and more effectively treats chronic diseases, which is critically important in the United States today because of the alarming rate of increase in diseases. For example, just 25 years ago Autism impacted one in 10,000 people. It now affects one in 65! This is a disturbing statistic that is preventable. How do we know this? If you look in history books, you'll find no reference to a condition that even sounds like autism to any significant degree until the dawn of the Industrial Revolution, when we began recklessly spewing toxins into our atmosphere.

The rate of chronic disease in children has increased from 12% to 30% over the past 20 years. As I previously stated, the *New England Journal of Medicine* reports that this generation of children is expected to have a shorter life expectancy than its parents. This may be the first generation not to outlive its parents in 200 years! Children are now officially paying for our poor lifestyle choices and our failure to protect them.

The time to act is now to reverse this unfathomable statistic. Thankfully our younger generations are aware of this and have already begun to swing the pendulum in the opposite direction starting with our Millennials, who are not comfortable following the status quo for its own sake! As Rumi stated 800 years ago "What's the use of old and frozen thought?" In this case, old and frozen thought is dangerous!

I explain in this book what I've learned as an integrative physician that helps explain the root causes of the rapid decline in our health despite our technological advances **AND *provide you with a roadmap to reclaim your health and wellbeing***. We can't solve a problem from the level of consciousness that created it. We must evolve and grow into a higher level of consciousness that already knows. This higher level of consciousness is achieved by **going within**, as ancient religious philosophies have advised for thousands of years. We call it FAITH.

I hope to inspire and empower millions of people to shift our paradigm to one of promoting wellness not only for ourselves, but for our children, who are the most important natural resource we have. I'll give you helpful tips to **F**earlessly **A**ffirm and **I**ntend to **T**ransform **H**ealth! Have FAITH and join me on the path to wellness!

CHAPTER TWO

IN THE BEGINNING

Nature Provides A Roadmap

Our species, now called Anatomically Modern Humans, appeared in a pre-existing environment with all the necessary tools for life, reproduction, and survival already at its disposal 200,000 years ago. Modern DNA analysis has revealed that our genetic code hasn't changed at all since we appeared on planet Earth. When an organism comes into existence, it seamlessly blends *into* its environment; it's part of its environment. Nature has it all figured out — if only we would listen. Nature provided the correct climate, lighting, and food for any organism to live and thrive. As we evolved, the foods that were naturally available to us were the foods we were supposed to eat to maintain a balanced life. Our climate was perfect for our survival and our reproduction. Even the number of hours of daylight are perfectly suited for us. The frequency of light from the sun at dawn and dusk heal our bodies! We're created to be in sync with the electromagnetic field of the planet, as studies have now confirmed! Being out of sync with this field due to stress and toxins, increases the risk of disease. Yes, we had predators and other threats 200,000 years ago, but we also had a system in place called "fight-or-flight" to protect us. Nature had this figured out, too. I often joke with my clients that if nature was relying on modern man to "fix" it with our x-ray machines, surgery and drugs, we'd have been extinct long ago!

What Would Nature Do?

When consistent changes occur to the environment, nature has built-in mechanisms called **evolution** to make permanent changes to the structure and function of organisms so they can once again live harmoniously in their environment and survive.

Complex evolution takes thousands, even millions, of years to happen. Mass extinctions happen due to abrupt changes in the environment, such as the meteor that struck the earth in New Mexico 65 million years ago and caused the majority of the species, most notably the dinosaurs on planet Earth, to go extinct. What we've experienced in the past one to two hundred years with man-made changes to our environment isn't equivalent to that infamous meteor strike, but it's so insidious we don't realize that we're gradually rendering our bodies extinct. Although many changes have provided tremendous advancement and advantage, those changes come at a heavy price — our health! We are the sickest wealthy country on the planet. And in our modern history, no single event has brought this to light more than the coronavirus pandemic that has taken the lives of hundreds of thousands of Americans as of the writing of this book. Countries with 3x our population have fewer cases and deaths from Coronavirus than we do. If these grim facts don't drive this point home, nothing else will. The Coronavirus pandemic has sharply brought to light the myths propagated by a broken medical system. The false claim that so many Americans are dying of Coronavirus because of lack of exposure to the virus is patently ridiculous and leaves out the most important branch of our immune system, which is called the **Innate** immune system. The idea that the only ways to acquire immunity are through vaccines or exposure to the microbe to prevent infection is a myth. Our bodies have innate, built-in immunity and can identify microbes that don't belong in the body and immediately destroy them **IF** the immune system is working properly. Numerous studies have shown that nutrient deficiencies greatly impair innate immunity and this is actually the main reason Americans have been so negatively impacted by Coronavirus. While this idea seems simplistic, you'll see why it's true as you proceed through this book. Gathering data on Coronavirus has certainly been challenging, but no matter how you slice this pie, we underperformed even on our best days. And contrary to popular belief, it's not because there aren't enough tests or access to testing. It's not because we didn't yet have a vaccine or blockbuster drug to treat it. It's simply because we've allowed our immunity to be destroyed by the stress, toxins, and drugs to which we've been exposed over the past century or more. About 100 years ago, the main cause of death throughout the world was infection. Rather than addressing its root cause, we created a pharmaceutical industry to synthesize antibiotics and vaccines. It took less than 80 years for these vaccines and antibiotics to run their course and today, we have significant antibiotic resistance and are seeing what are being called "superbugs" that plow their way through all antibiotics and their victims. Scrambling to make vaccines against every bug that causes significant infection is like another game of "whack-a-mole," yet we continue to react with the same knee jerk responses with no consideration of why our innate immunity isn't working as anticipated. Instead, we rush to circumvent the problem after thousands have died. The pharmaceutical industry has run out of ideas about what new antibiotics to make because the faster they make them, the faster the bugs seem to become resistant. It's a frightening prospect to think that infection may once again become the main cause of death throughout the world just like it was just a century ago despite the arsenal of technology, antibiotics, and vaccines we've amassed.

What if malnutrition was the actual reason we're so susceptible to the average bug and to so many diseases? I'll demonstrate throughout this book why the restoration of our immune systems and body functions to the way *nature* originally designed them is critical to our wellbeing. I'll discuss the studies that show that nutrient deficits of vitamins A, C, D, folate, zinc, iron, selenium and copper reduce our innate ability to fight infections.

Science is showing that we should be living about 120 years based on the examination of telomeres, which are the ends of chromosomes that keep them healthy for cell division and lifespan. Why haven't we reached this mark with all this technology? In fact, our life expectancy has declined for the past 2 out of 3 years according to the CDC. Why is our life expectancy actually declining rather than rising like other countries in the world?

Did you know that 50% of Americans are expected to acquire a chronic disease before age 18 or that more than 80% of Americans suffer from more than one disease by age 65? People are consistently reporting unprecedented stress in their lives like never before, and as I mentioned earlier, autism now affects one in 65!

These alarming statistics are mostly due to abrupt man-made environmental changes, but we can *reverse the impact*. Modern changes that adversely affect the well-being of the population include:

- the use of pesticides on crops which destroys its delicate balance of microbes and nutrients.

- the implementation of rapid farming that strips minerals from our soil.
- the consumption of genetically modified foods.
- the use of radiation.
- the ingestion of processed foods.
- the ingestion of pasturized foods.
- the feeding of hormones and antibiotics to livestock and poultry.
- farm-raising of fish
- the overuse of antibiotics.
- exposure to dangerous electromagnetic fields from devices like cell phones, laptops, wifi, and televisions
- the use of synthetic prescription and over-the-counter drugs.
- the use of household toxins mascarading as cleaning products and personal hygiene products.
- the widespread production and use of plastics.
- the exposure to artificial light.
- changing the molecular structure of water with chemical processing

Even some gender role changes have occurred which create stressors in our lives. I'll cover this topic later. All of these man-made changes happened faster than the human body could evolve and this is the main reason these man-made changes have been so destructive. *It's important to distinguish evolution from adaptation.* These man-made changes caused the body to **adapt** on the fly to make adjustments to insure immediate survival. This shouldn't be mistaken as evolution. Evolution helps assure long-term survival by changing the structure and function of the body through its DNA (genes); but adaptation is more short-term and may not be effective long-term. So while an organism may be able to *adapt* short-term, this can come at a heavy price. These changes the body has to make to survive cause symptoms such as fatigue, weight gain, sleep disturbances, weakened immunity, anxiety, and depression. Left unchecked, these symptoms progress to diseases such as heart disease, cancer, stroke, Alzheimer's dementia, and many other conditions. And if we take a hard look at our current coronavirus crisis, we'll see the real reasons we've been so much more severely impacted than other countries.

According to the International Agency for Research on Cancer, we're exposed to more than 100 chemicals known to cause cancer in humans, otherwise known as carcinogens! We're also exposed to 75 additional toxins labeled as *probably* carcinogenic to humans. It's estimated that we're exposed to over 200 different known toxins before we even leave our homes in the morning! And the list is growing fast. There are well over 80,000 chemicals in production and only 2,000 have actually been studied. It's very likely that many of the remaining 78,000 unstudied chemicals are toxic and may cause cancer, but it'll be years, if not decades, before this information is available.

A study conducted by the Environmental Working Group in 2005 tested umbilical cord blood in newborn infants and found 281 chemicals circulating in the cord blood of developing babies! 180 of them are known to cause cancer in humans or animals. We once thought the placenta shielded developing infants from toxins, but this study proved this is not the case. *These chemical exposures are significant causes of autism and childhood cancer*. The risk of these diseases is not linked to genes, but to the toxins and damage they cause before our children are even born. The evidence for this link is mounting. Mount Sinai in N.Y.C. released a study in May 2017 linking the exposure of babies to toxins in late pregnancy and early life to the risk of autism. In October 2013, the American College of Obstetricians and Gynecologists released a committee opinion which stated the following: "The evidence that links exposure to toxic environmental agents and adverse reproductive and developmental health outcomes is sufficiently robust, and the American College of Obstetricians and Gynecologists and the American Society for Reproductive Medicine join leading scientists and other clinical practitioners in calling for timely action to identify and reduce exposure to toxic environmental agents while addressing the consequences of such exposure."

This committee opinion also states the following: "Prenatal exposure to certain chemicals has been documented to increase the risk of cancer in childhood; adult male exposure to pesticides is linked to altered semen quality, sterility, and prostate cancer; and postnatal exposure to some pesticides can interfere with all developmental stages of reproductive function in adult females, including puberty, menstruation and ovulation, fertility and fecundity, and menopause."

Data is now emerging to suggest that experiences in the womb have consequences for generations! A study published by the University of Cambridge in March 2011 showed that a gene called Hnf4a is influenced by diet. This gene is involved in the development of the pancreas and later production of insulin by the pancreas. Hnf4a is known to be present in both rats and humans. Cambridge University studied rats and gave the mothers a poor diet consisting of low protein during their pregnancies. This resulted in the loss of the function of the Hnf4a gene in the offspring rats *resulting in higher rates of type 2 diabetes later in life*. Rats whose mothers didn't eat poorly during pregnancy didn't have this result. The study of the DNA revealed that **this gene was specifically impacted by environmental factors** consisting of poor diet in this case. We call this epigenetic. When this gene was studied in humans, it was shown that this same gene is also responsible for the same functions in humans and presumably, the same mechanism is involved in human children whose mothers eat poorly during pregnancy! **This study is critically important because it shows that genes do not determine our fate, but lifestyle choices**

do! In the case of developing fetuses, our mom's choices may determine our fate not because our mom may give us bad genes, but because perfectly normal genes get damaged by poor food choices.

A study published in the *Journal of Reproductive Toxicology* reported that exposure to arsenic, tobacco smoke, air pollutants and hormone-disrupting toxins while still in the womb are well established as causes of disease later in life. In some cases, the grandchildren are even impacted - that's *two generations impacted.*

A well-studied example is the risk of otherwise rare cervical cancers known as adenocarcinoma of the cervix in the daughters **and granddaughters** of women exposed to the *synthetic* estrogen, DES (diethylstilbestrol), used in the 1940s and 50s to treat certain pregnancy complications. The drug was subsequently banned, but its negative impact can still be felt over 70 years later!

Unborn children exposed to arsenic are at increased risk of lung cancer and other lung diseases, certain skin lesions, and bladder cancers. The link has been directly associated to damage to genes caused by arsenic. This doesn't mean that it's genetic, this means it's *epigenetic* and there's a huge difference. **Epigenetic means otherwise normal genes that can be damaged by environmental influences. Genetic means it's fixed and unchangeable regardless of environmental influences.**

Unborn children exposed to tobacco smoke have increased risk of premature birth, cancer, diabetes, asthma and other lung diseases through damage to previously normal genes.

The *Journal of Reproductive Toxicology* also reported on a group of 100 chemicals called benzopyrenes and PAHs (polycyclic aromatic hydrocarbons). These toxins are released through the burning of coal, tobacco, trash, wood, oil and gasoline. Unborn children exposed to these toxic chemicals have increased risk of lower IQ, developmental delay, low birth weight, and behavioral disorders. These chemicals resemble steroid hormones and are called hormone disruptors because they abnormally bind to cells and prevent the real hormones from functioning. Hormones are critical because they help determine what genes are turned on and off. I'll discuss hormones in more detail in chapter 15.

Finally, the *Journal of Reproductive Toxicology* also reported on phthalates, which comprise a large group of chemicals found in most homes as they are found in glues, building materials, personal care products, medical devices, detergents, packaging, children's toys, pharmaceutical medications, food products, and textiles. Unborn children exposed to these chemicals are at increased risk of developmental defects such as abnormal neurological development in girls and undescended testes in boys. Phthalates are also considered hormone disruptors as they look like hormones and bind abnormally to cells *preventing real hormones from functioning.* I'll explain later in this book just how critical our hormones are to our body function.

In the next chapter I'll discuss how these man-made changes have led us to our current healthcare crisis and how we can begin to regain our health through better understanding and a better paradigm that seeks to restore wellness using systems of medicine better equipped than our own to tackle this crisis.

CHAPTER THREE

SHORTCUTS OR SHORT CIRCUITS?

In an effort to help people who have symptoms of fatigue, weight gain, or chronic diseases feel better, we often inadvertently create more problems in allopathic medicine. For example, medication to treat heartburn causes thinning of the bones, called osteoporosis. Medication to treat high cholesterol has been found to increase the risk of diabetes and even kidney failure. Medications prescribed for anxiety, as well as medications for managing pain, are highly addictive and have been shown in studies to cause almost irreversible structural changes in the brain. Some anti-inflammatory medications have been shown to increase the risk of heart attacks and strokes, and some have even been removed from the market such as Vioxx®, which was abruptly withdrawn in 2004 due to safety concerns. We also now know that anti-inflammatory medications actually prevent the body from healing and further damage our joints.

The concept of medications was a good one in theory, but where did we go wrong? There are two principle problems with prescription drugs. First, while the concept of medicines originated with plants, their active ingredients were sought in a lab, concentrated, and given to people. The problem with this approach is that one concentrated ingredient is rarely safe long-term.

In Chinese medicine and many other natural systems of medicine, the quality of an entire plant is known and kept intact. This minimizes side effects. It's known in Chinese medicine that a single herb may have toxicity, so Chinese herbal formulas consist of multiple herbs and include specific herbs that counter the toxicity in order to provide a more balanced correction of a problem without side effects. For example, if an herb can cause dryness as a side effect, another herb that moistens is added to maintain balance.

Antidepressants such as SSRIs (Selective Serotonin Reuptake Inhibitors) are used to treat depression in allopathic medicine. The single active ingredient in one such SSRI is fluoxetine. Fluoxetine and other antidepressants are known to have some potentially serious side effects. In addition to side effects and adverse reactions, the actual treatment can backfire and cause worse depression than the patient had before the medication was started. Antidepressants are particularly dangerous in children and adolescents. In fact, the FDA released a formal warning about SSRIs stating that there is a risk of suicide with their use in children.

POTENTIAL FLUOXETINE SIDE EFFECTS

Suicide, worsening of depression, mania, serotonin syndrome (possible life threatening increase of serotonin), low sodium, excessive urination due to anti-diuretic hormone release from the brain (leading to dehydration known as SIADH), seizures, low blood sugar, allergic reaction, abnormal heart rhythms, abnormal bleeding due to effect on bone marrow (leading to low platelets), low blood pressure, glaucoma, a skin condition called erythema multiforme, and pulmonary fibrosis.

In allopathic medicine, depression is diagnosed using the DSM-V (Diagnostic and Statistical Manual of Mental Disorders) criteria which lists a series of signs and symptoms to clinically diagnose depression. Once diagnosed, a patient is prescribed medication and/or therapy.

TCM evaluates the causes of depression *energetically* by determining the patterns of disharmony or root causes present in each client to prescribe a customized formula that suits their particular patterns. There are about 12 patterns of disharmony that cause depression according to TCM theory. After proper diagnosis of the root cause or pattern of disharmony, a custom herbal formula is prescribed. An example of such a formula is Xiao Yao San (Free and Easy Wanderer), which is used for a pattern called "Liver *qi* (pronounced *chee*) stagnation against a background of liver blood deficiency."

FORMULA FOR XIAO YAO SAN

This formula consists of eight herbs:

- •Bo He (Peppermint) (3 grams)
- •Chai Hu (dried Bupleurum root) (9 grams)
- •Dang Gui (Angelica root) (9 grams)
- •Bai Shao (White Peony root) (12 grams)
- •Bai Zhu (White Atractylodes rhizome) (9 grams)
- •Fu ling (Poria) (15 grams)
- •Gan cao (Licorice root) (6 grams)
- •Sheng jiang (Fresh ginger rhizome) (3 slices)

Rather than using just one herb, which would likely cause side effects, a balanced formula is composed that matches the pattern of disharmony causing the depression. Xiao Yao San was shown in a meta-analysis study done in 2012 published by the journal *Evidence Based Complementary and Alternative Medicine,* to be just as effective as antidepressants when properly used for the right pattern of liver *qi* stagnation against a background of liver blood deficiency. It's also been shown in studies to have far fewer side effects and to be extremely well-tolerated. What's critical to know about TCM is that the formula MUST match the pattern of disharmony in order to work with minimal or no side effects. Diagnosis is critical in TCM.

Another amazing example comes from the *Journal of Allergy and Immunology*, who published a study by Mount Sinai and the University of Beijing in 2005 which showed that a Chinese herbal formula they called ASHMI (Anti-asthma herbal medication intervention) was as effective as the powerful steroid Prednisone® for the treatment of asthma *without the side effects of Prednisone®*. The herbal formula also corrected abnormally low cortisol levels noted in the children with asthma. Long-term or repeated use of the drug

Prednisone® damages the adrenal system initially increasing, then permanently lowering, cortisol below normal levels. Prednisone® can cause diabetes, immune suppression, and weight gain. The Chinese herb which was shown to be just as effective as Prednisone® has been extensively studied by Mount Sinai for over 17 years with no side effects! It's also been used in TCM for thousands of years.

The second issue with medications is that most of them are synthetic or artificial. Nature isn't designed to deal with synthetic drugs, and our bodies are no different. We evolved in our environment to deal with the things that were present in our environment at the time. Man has created so many synthetic toxins that our bodies are now overwhelmed with them as we discussed in chapter two.

The organ known as the liver is principally responsible for processing and eliminating medications and other toxins from the body's blood stream, but the liver is running into difficulty processing unnatural things. Medical studies show that this causes vitamin, mineral, and enzyme deficiencies that cause symptoms we recognize as the side effects to many drugs, such as fluoxetine and Prednisone® sited above. When the liver isn't functioning properly, toxic build-up creates inflammation. This inflammation spills into the rest of the body and into our cells, which creates the symptoms that we experience as medication side effects.

Prevention of Death or Disease?

What we call prevention in allopathic medicine isn't really prevention. Why is that? When we speak of *prevention* in allopathic medicine, we're referring to having a physical exam and obtaining mammograms and colonoscopies, for example. These tests clearly don't prevent diseases. Mammograms are used for the early diagnosis of breast cancer, and colonoscopies are used for the early diagnosis of colon cancer. So, they really are methods for *early diagnosis*, not prevention. They catch things early and prevent death, not disease. We must face the alarming realization that our current healthcare paradigm is the *prevention of death.* It must become *prevention of disease,* and more importantly, the ***promotion of wellness.***

Why Early Detection Isn't Good Enough

While early detection is better than nothing, it's not good enough. It's always best not to get a particular condition than to have to treat it at all and endure the symptoms, erosion of health, and psychological trauma that ensues.

The alarming number of diseases we face today is unprecedented, and that number has increased in a very short period of time. People often use the flawed explanation that we have more diseases because we're living longer. The fact that more children have adult-onset diseases than ever before proves clearly that this problem is not one of aging! Childhood cancer is also on the rise, obviously not because our children are getting older! Age-matched comparisons between Americans and people in other developed nations also proves this is not the case.

The National Institutes of Health released a report in 2011 that revealed the life expectancy for men and women in the United States was **last** among the ten richest countries in the world. For men over 50, the life expectancy in the United States increased 2.5 years over the past 25 years. The life expectancy for the same demographic group in Japan increased 6.4 years! In Italy the life expectancy grew 5.9 years. Although we believe our life expectancy has significantly increased, it has grown far slower than all other wealthy nations in the world despite the fact that we spend far more money on our health! And to add insult to injury, our life expectancy here in the U.S. has actually been dropping for 2 out of the past 3 years according to the CDC. Getting older is clearly not the reason for these daunting statistics we see today.

The reason for this slow increase and recent drop in life expectancy is the alarming number of chronic diseases that Americans experience, often before they even hit age 18! The concerning **deterioration in our health can be reversed**, however. It's not necessary to be diagnosed with a chronic disease when there are time-proven methods and cutting-edge technology available today that are very affordable and, in fact, cheaper than the conventional diagnostic methods we currently use. *Holistic or integrative methods can find the root cause of symptoms long before they become diseases and correct them.*

Treating a disease is always more expensive than preventing it, and sometimes the improper treatment of diseases causes other diseases. The average cost in the United States per chronic disease exceeds $7,000 per year by the latest estimates. The total annual U.S. cost of cancer care is projected to reach $175 billion by 2020, an increase of 40 percent from 2010. The U.S. spends much more than any other country, even the entire *continent* of Europe, on cancer care with marginal improvements. Population-adjusted data reveals the U.S. experiences 729,000 more deaths annually due to cancer than Europe and spends $1.6 billion more than Europe for cancer care annually.

The chemotherapy used to treat cancer is not only expensive in cost but can increase the risk of other cancers and other diseases later on, while having minimal impacts on the primary cancer. The side effects of many cancer treatments can be disabling, causing fatigue, hair loss, life-threatening infections, gastrointestinal issues, nerve damage, and much more. Cancer treatments are also linked to more than double the risk of heart disease. This type of suffering is no longer needed. Why go through all that if you don't have to?

The Milken Foundation produced a report in 2007 called "An Unhealthy America" and projected that just modest preventive care can increase the GDP (gross domestic product), which is an economic indicator, by 18% in approximately 40 years. That's six trillion dollars back into the economy with just modest preventive strategies. A follow-up report by the Milken Foundation called "Checkup Time" released in 2014 showed that we had made little to no progress toward this goal. Why? Our allopathic medical system is failing because it's not designed for prevention or to promote wellness.

Why Treatment Based on Symptoms Is Flawed

A premise of allopathic medicine is to treat symptoms as a basis of treating disease. For example, a patient I'll call Jane went to the emergency room one night with severe chest pain. The ER doctor evaluated Jane and found no signs of a heart attack or other life-threatening condition. The ER doctor diagnosed heartburn and prescribed an antacid. Jane followed up with her primary care physician, who referred her to a gastroenterologist, who found nothing wrong with her after performing an upper endoscopy which is a diagnostic test that looks for ulcers, masses, bleeding, and cancer. Allopathic testing isn't designed to look for the cause of symptoms, so all the testing done for Jane was normal. The doctor's recommendation was for her to keep taking the antacid to treat the symptom of heartburn. Jane stayed on her antacid to mask the signs of her pain for years.

While this seems logical on the surface, traditional Chinese medical theory tells us that it's significantly flawed. In TCM, the emphasis is on balance of *yin* and *yang* or *life energies and essence, which means that the underlying cause should always be treated* and not just the symptoms.

If someone like Jane has heartburn and the treatment is specifically targeting that symptom without looking at the cause, the symptom simply recurs or spirals into another symptom – there's no balance achieved in this type of treatment. In TCM, the root cause of the symptom has to be successfully treated in order for the symptom to go away. The symptom doesn't go away because it's masked, but because balance is restored in the body. The root cause must be treated not just so the symptoms go away, but also so the condition doesn't get worse.

When Jane first came to see me, she was tired all the time, still had the heartburn when she tried to stop her antacid, and was developing other symptoms such as aches and pains in her muscles and joints, which she didn't have before starting her antacid. I evaluated her according to TCM principles and noted that she had spleen qi deficiency, accumulation of damp, and toxic heat, which would be the rough equivalent of a weak metabolism, inflammation, and acidity in allopathic medicine. It's important to point out here that organs in TCM are not anatomical organs as we understand them, but are *energy fields* which have specific functions. I'll discuss TCM in more detail in chapter 7.

I prescribed a specific nutritional plan for Jane to treat the toxic heat and damp. Jane immediately started a dairy and wheat-free, raw, alkaline diet, and I performed tests for her to determine what her specific deficiencies were. I also looked for the source of her toxic heat, which was causing her heartburn; this turned out to be a small intestine bacterial overgrowth (SIBO), which we successfully treated with natural methods. Jane had ten different nutrient deficiencies in vitamins, minerals, and antioxidants which was weakening her immunity and causing build-up of more inflammation and acidity. This inflammation was causing her joint and muscle pains. Her fatigue was caused by the significant number of nutrient deficits she had. We corrected them with nutrition and supplements. Jane's energy was much better, and she no longer required antacids after a few months of treatment. She's been able to maintain her good health with a maintenance plan which actively promotes her wellness. Her nutrition plan changed as her patterns of disharmony improved to one that was less restrictive and more balanced. Continuing a restrictive diet past its utility would produce other imbalances and should be avoided according to TCM.

Jane is an excellent example of why taking antacids for heartburn rarely works to successfully treat the heartburn pain. It simply comes back once the medication is stopped and leads to other complications down the road. Studies are showing that the long-term use of antacids is related to bone deterioration (osteoporosis) and most recently kidney dysfunction because the antacids block absorption of critical nutrients into the body.

Balance is the key in traditional Chinese medicine, so if something is too high or too low, a symptom can result. Hot flashes are a great example. Hot flashes are often due to high or low levels of estrogen, but sometimes they aren't due to estrogen at all. Sometimes hot flashes are caused by high cortisol, excessive thyroid hormone levels, heavy metals, or other toxins accumulating in the body. If hot flashes are treated solely based on the symptom, the problem would not be successfully resolved even if the hot flashes go away.

I'll call the next patient Mary to protect her identity. When Mary came to the office, she was taking hormones prescribed elsewhere for severe hot flashes after having a hysterectomy. When her hot flashes didn't improve, her doctor increased the dose of her estrogen, but her symptoms persisted. I evaluated Mary based on TCM theory and determined that she had patterns of damp retention and spleen-kidney deficiency. Kidney in TCM is significantly different than what we recognize as kidney in allopathic medicine. According to TCM, this meant, in part, that Mary's reserve energy, essence, and hormone reserves were very low, and she was retaining a lot of fluid in her body. I surmised that the fluid retention was due to estrogen dominance as Mary was only prescribed estrogen, as is customary in allopathic medicine following a hysterectomy. One of estrogen's numerous functions is to hold on to water in the body. That's one of the reasons balancing estrogen with progesterone is important regardless of whether you've had a hysterectomy. The human body is 99% water by molecule. In other words, 99% of all the molecules in your body are water molecules! Another way of saying this is that the body is 70% water by weight. So, it's clear that water metabolism is critical to body function and just because someone's uterus was removed doesn't mean that she no longer requires proper balance and proper water metabolism. I'll discuss hormones in more detail in chapter 15.

Given the TCM patterns, we proceeded with hormone and nutrient testing. Test results revealed that the estrogen levels in her cells were way too high, and she had very little progesterone to balance estrogen, making her extremely estrogen dominant. That was the reason for her hot flashes and water retention. I switched Mary to bio-identical hormones, reduced her estrogen dose, and added progesterone. Her adrenal glands were also depleted due to chronic stress, so I prescribed herbs to support her adrenals, along with DHEA and testosterone because these important adrenal hormones were also quite low. Mary's hot flashes were much less severe when she came in for follow-up the next month. Had I used Mary's symptoms alone to treat her, I would never have known which hormones she needed. In her case, treating the adrenals was critical because she was also feeling tired and gaining weight after her surgery. Mary's nutrition testing revealed 13 nutrient deficits which we corrected with oral supplementation. Blood work didn't reveal these deficiencies, but cellular-based testing did. This is because symptoms arise from the cells, not the blood stream. It's the abnormal cellular function that leads to the onset of symptoms, so if we don't look in the right place, we don't get the answers we need. We encouraged and guided Mary in looking at her stressful lifestyle to make some important changes as well as practice mindfulness meditation and take time for herself.

Another glaring example of a shortcut that's a short circuit is the injudicious use of antibiotics. For life-threatening conditions, antibiotics are absolutely necessary to prevent death; however, we have used antibiotics for too many unnecessary reasons, such as colds, acne, rashes, and viral infections. The use of antibiotics in these cases is not only needless but dangerous long term. We're now seeing significant resistance to antibiotics due to this injudicious use. The development of "superbugs" has been reported since 2002, but has now become a major health concern according to the World Health Organization. This has spawned a desperate search for treatments for resistant infections and guess where they're looking? They're asking mother nature for cures now that the synthetic and artificial cesspool has been exhausted. Modern antibiotics were discovered by Alexander Fleming 80 years ago, when he discovered penicillin. This spawned the pharmaceutical industry and the push for artificial and synthetic drugs began. Due to this reckless pursuit of profit, we're in a health crisis with 1.5 million projected deaths in Europe alone by 2050 due to "superbugs."

Thankfully, mother nature has a forgiving nature. A paper published in the journal *Critical Care* in October 2018 postulated that a life-threatening infection called sepsis could be successfully treated using IV high dose vitamin C, hydrocortisone and the vitamin thiamin.

This paper used what's already known in human physiology as well as preliminary studies already done to show promise for a more natural treatment for even the most life-threatening of infections. This paper was sparked by the brave decision of Dr. Paul Marik, a critical care specialist in Norfolk, Virginia, who used this modality on 700 patients dying in the intensive care unit of his hospital. They made what were thought to be miraculous recoveries with no side effects! Sepsis is a potentially fatal infection that spreads to the blood stream (also called blood poisoning). One in five people affected by sepsis die from this condition even with early treatment with antibiotics. It's the leading cause of non-cardiac death in intensive care settings. Several larger studies are taking place to further test the idea that the natural agents, IV vitamin C, thiamin and hydrocortisone can reverse this deadly condition without side effects.

The CITRIS-ALI study released in the *Journal of the American Medical Association* in January 2020, showed that high dose IV vitamin C reduced mortality and ICU-free days in patients suffering from sepsis. This study has served as the basis for some hospitals to use high dose IV vitamin C to combat the coronavirus pandemic.

A second monumental study that didn't get as much attention was published in 2018 by the journal *Frontiers of Microbiology*. This study looked at the folk medicine of Northern Ireland where components of grass and soil were used by the Druids to cure toothaches, throat and neck infections over a thousand years ago. To their astonishment, a strain of bacteria called Streptomyces was found in this grass and soil. This bacterium produces a natural antibiotic to defend itself against other bugs, and this natural antibiotic was effective against four of the six "superbugs" tested including MRSA (methicillin-resistant staphylococcus aureus and VRE (vancomycin-resistant enterococcus).

Upper respiratory infections are most frequently caused by viruses and patients report feeling better after using antibiotics. This isn't because the antibiotic killed the virus. Antibiotics help reduce superficial inflammation and therefore *appear* to help certain conditions when, in fact, the problem isn't related to a bacterial infection at all, which is what antibiotics treat. It's because antibiotics are "cooling" according to TCM and give the impression of working because they reduce the inflammation with their cooling properties, but leave the virus alive in the body for the patient's own immunity to combat. Antibiotics don't kill viruses or yeast. In fact, they're more likely to promote yeast infections due to the destruction of the good bacteria that usually keep yeast in check. ***Antibiotics also set up the next infection by weakening the immune system***. This is why we increasingly see patients being treated with multiple rounds of antibiotics for a cold that seems to linger for weeks. While antibiotics appear to reduce inflammation short term, the inflammation returns with a vengeance due to a weakened immune system leading the patient and their doctors to think that the infection is still raging. Breaking this cycle with more natural immune-boosting agents is critical during this time. Traditional Chinese medicine, as we'll explore in the later chapters, has a very profound and comprehensive understanding of the immune system and provides highly effective natural herbal remedies for upper respiratory infections of different types with minimal to no side effects while building immunity and preventing future infections. A client I'll call Joe was referred to me by his wife because he had been treated with three different rounds of antibiotics for a "cold" that lingered for over almost two months. He had a dry cough that kept him up at night and he had alternating fever and chills. His doctor prescribed multiple antibiotics, prednisone® (a powerful artificial steroid) and an inhaler. Joe would feel better for a few days then relapse. His blood work and chest x-ray were normal. My assessment of Joe revealed that he was no longer infectious but the pathogen (likely a virus) was buried deeper in his body in what is known as the shao yang layer in TCM. He was also suffering from lung dryness due to the inflammation and heat produced by the viral infection. I prescribed a Chinese herbal formula for Joe and made recommendations for probiotics to replenish his bacterial flora. Joe felt much better in a few days and didn't relapse this time. We then worked on his immune system to build it up to protect him in the future. I advised him to avoid antibiotics and steroids for common colds and recommended he take more natural agents as soon as he suspected a cold and seek the care of an integrative physician *first* to assess the possibility of using natural agents rather than further damaging his immune system with antibiotics and artificial steroids.

TCM theory is based on treating the underlying root cause of symptoms rather than masking them with medications. *TCM also provides a roadmap instructing us how to identify and treat these root causes.* This isn't possible with our allopathic medical system. There are critical reasons why this is important. In the next chapter, I'll review how the body has unseen forces that are always surveilling and promoting the most efficient path for proper body function. I call these self-correcting forces. It's the way the body heals itself *if given the opportunity*. When we mask symptoms with medications, we prevent the body's self-correcting forces from working, and more problems develop later. Jane, Mary, and Joe are valuable examples of this principle that I'll explain in the next chapter.

CHAPTER FOUR

SELF-CORRECTING FORCES

The human body has built-in correcting forces we don't understand, but they work every time *as long as the body has the right tools at its disposal to make it happen*. Our hearts beat over and over again, day after day, decade after decade without our conscious intervention. In fact, our hearts beat 115,000 times a day. If we had to think about our hearts beating, we wouldn't live very long, would we? When we cut our skin, it heals and looks like new in no time without our conscious intervention. If we have a significant zinc deficiency and we cut ourselves, it may not heal so well. If we have a CoQ10 deficiency, our muscles can get inflamed and we may experience pain.

The body has to maintain a relationship with its environment because it's part of its environment. It's becoming increasingly clear based on sound scientific data that the environment is more important for gene expression and function than the genes themselves! What I mean by environment is the macro-environment we see around us, as well as the micro-environment inside the cells themselves. While genes are responsible for the myriad of proteins the body makes to maintain its physical structure and execute body function, the condition of the ***environment*** where the genes are located inside the cells is the critical factor that determines which genes get turned on or off. This same *environment is also a critical factor in determining if those genes in the body's cells get damaged* by toxins!

A foundational premise of TCM is that the body is constantly communicating with the environment in order to maintain balance. TCM understands this relationship well. This ability of the body to communicate with the environment allows the body to make critical decisions related to survival.

Cells are the body's basic building blocks. We have between 70 *trillion* to 100 *trillion* cells in the body working tirelessly day and night to make energy to power our body functions. Energy-based medical systems recognize this and provide evaluations and treatments to take this critical fact into account. Figure 1 illustrates the genetic information housed in each of our cells.

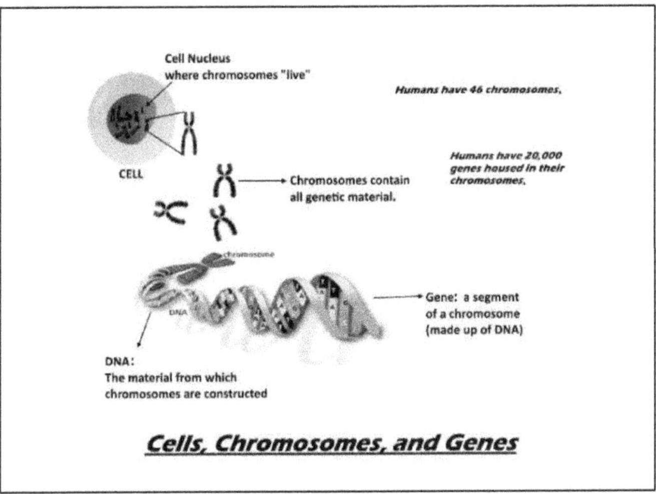

Figure 1: Human cells have 46 chromosomes. There are about 25,000 genes housed in these 46 chromosomes. Each gene is made of DNA (deoxyribonucleic acid). Genes are proteins, which serve as blueprints for cellular function. Genes are turned on or off by hormones.

According to Dr. Craig Venter, a pioneer in genomic research, "Human biology is actually far more complicated than we imagine. Everybody talks about the genes that they received from their mother and father, for this trait or the other. But in reality, those genes have very little impact on life outcomes. Our biology is way too complicated for that and deals with hundreds of thousands of independent factors. Genes are absolutely not our fate. They can give us useful information about the increased risk of a disease, but in most cases, they will not determine the actual cause of the disease, or the actual incidence of somebody getting it. Most biology will come from the complex interaction of all the proteins and cells working with environmental factors, not driven directly by the genetic code."

This quote by Dr. Venter is critical. He's stating in no uncertain terms that genes are not, in most cases, the cause of disease. This premise has stood up to the rigors of science, too. No matter how we slice the disease pie, whether we're looking at Alzheimer's dementia, autism, heart disease or cancer, only approximately 3-5% of cases are directly caused by genes. Figure 2 illustrates the distribution of the causes of disease.

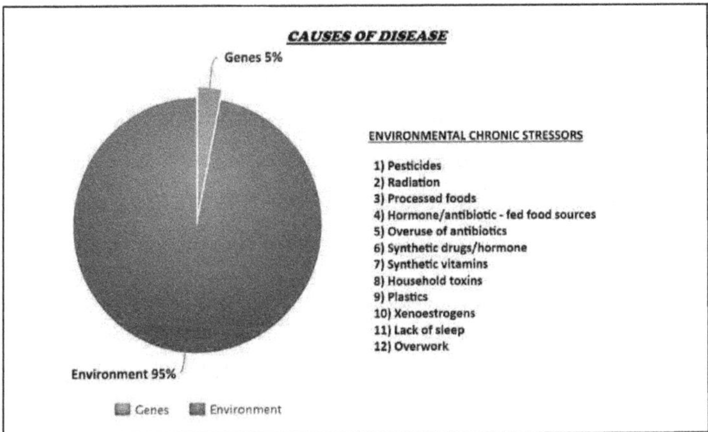

Figure 2: This illustration demonstrates the percentage of diseases attributable to genes vs. environment. 5% of diseases are directly genetically-based. The remaining 95% are caused by the environment of the cell, not its genes. These environmental factors can lead to gene damage over time, leading us to believe the diseases are genetic when they are environmental in nature.

Between Normal and Disease — The Gray Zone

When I was training as an allopathic physician, I was taught to diagnose and treat diseases. This knowledge was valuable when helping people who had acute life-threatening diseases, such as appendicitis, which can be fatal. Now a simple surgical procedure helps save lives every day so allopathic medicine is extremely important. It helps us diagnose and treat acute life-threatening conditions and saves countless lives.

We had patients with ectopic pregnancies, which are dangerous pregnancies that occur outside the uterus, most commonly in the fallopian tubes. While this condition continues to be fatal today, if it's diagnosed early enough, it can be treated medically or surgically, thanks to allopathic medicine, which has done a tremendous amount of good in preventing death from acute life-threatening conditions.

What I soon learned, though, was that allopathic medicine was not so good for healing chronic conditions and even worse at preventing them. I was trained to believe that if bloodwork and test results were within the *normal* range and there was no diagnosable disease present, there was nothing wrong.

My patients insisted, however, that they didn't feel good despite normal blood work and diagnostic testing. They continued to complain of fatigue, depression, and anxiety. They continued to grumble about a lack of sex drive and stubborn weight gain. I continued to do bloodwork and run other diagnostic tests, only to find nothing out of the ordinary. I kept assuring them everything was okay. For some patients, I recommended that they should take antidepressants, anxiety medications, or sleeping pills.

As I progressed in my practice and learned traditional Chinese medicine, it dawned on me that there was a "gray zone" that is invisible with bloodwork. In other words, what is considered to be a "normal" reference range in the lab is not, in fact, normal. As my thinking became more holistic and began to integrate all that I learned from allopathic medicine, traditional Chinese medicine, and functional medicine, I began to piece this puzzle together. Just because testing didn't diagnose a disease didn't mean all was normal. It just meant that the condition was not yet visible in the blood stream or with diagnostic testing!

When I began studying traditional Chinese medicine, it was necessary for me to literally forget all that I knew about allopathic medicine so I could allow the principles of Chinese medicine to sink in. They were so different. I had to develop a "beginner's mind." Beginner's mind is a Buddhist principle that is now being touted in the latest research as a learner's mind. It's a principle of suspending old ideas to allow new ones the space to develop.

At first, I wondered if TCM would ever make sense to me. The principles of TCM were so different than everything I'd been taught in medical school, and one day it all came together and opened up my mind like never before. Before I knew it, my medical and personal philosophies blended together perfectly, and everything made sense.

Your body's number one job is to keep you alive! Since the blood stream provides nutrients and oxygen to the heart, lungs, and brain, the body *tenaciously protects the blood stream to keep you alive*. If your blood doesn't have enough oxygen, hormones, vitamins, minerals, antioxidants, and other critical nutrients to properly feed the heart and brain, you could have a heart attack or stroke. Because the body is self-correcting, it can adjust the bloodstream to keep it normal. *And that is the reason so many people with nagging chronic symptoms have normal blood tests*. The body's activating a survival mechanism to make sure it gets blood to the heart and brain! This is how the body adapts to not having enough resources for all its cells and body functions. These are the self-correcting forces of the body at work! This survival tactic comes at a price that the body is willing to pay: fatigue, weight gain, depression, anxiety, low sex drive, memory loss, aches and pains, and more. These nagging symptoms are not immediately life-threatening like heart attacks and strokes are. These nagging symptoms linger if not corrected and can progress to more significant diseases like Alzheimer's dementia, diabetes, arthritis, cancer, weakened immunity, and more. Once you're diagnosed with these more serious diseases, you're no longer in the gray zone. Now your blood work and diagnostic studies are abnormal, but it's too late to prevent disease. Your body is still willing to pay this priced over a heart attack or stroke because none of those chronic diseases such as Alzheimer's dementia, diabetes, infection or even cancer is *immediately* life-threatening. If you have a heart attack, your body thinks you'll be dead now. If you get cancer, your body knows you won't be dead now – death may come at an undefined later time which it's willing to accept rather than dying now. Your body doesn't know that there are life-saving drastic medical maneuvers that can save your life even when you have a heart attack so it behaves accordingly to protect you almost at any other cost.

When self-correcting forces are activated, you barely notice at first. For example, our bones are a great source of minerals such as calcium, phosphorus, selenium, and magnesium. When there aren't enough of these minerals in the body, the body's self-correcting forces take these minerals from the skeletal bones to take to higher priority systems such as the brain and heart, resulting in osteoporosis (brittle bones). Your body will accept osteoporosis any day over a heart attack! In traditional Chinese medicine, there's a term for this called *inter-transformation.* Why would the body do this? It turns out that the body has built-in corrective forces because it anticipates that supplies might be low at times. Nature thought of everything! If it didn't have this flexibility, we'd be extinct by now.

The unprecedented stress and toxins we experience today cause chronic deficiencies in nutrients, hormones, enzymes and other necessary factors that fuel body function. Your body's self-correcting mechanisms know that if your bloodstream can't carry oxygen and blood to the organs that keep you alive, you will die. It does everything it can to help you survive. And all this is going on in plain sight once we change to a perception that allows us to see it. As we hurriedly go through our day, we don't really listen deeply to the early signs. The early warnings are your nagging symptoms and signs: fatigue, weight gain, depression, anxiety, insomnia, aches and pains, etc.

Your body will self-correct until it literally cannot do so anymore, leading to diseases. It's a simple matter of supply and demand. The more demand there is, the more likely there will be a shortage of supply. If the supply/demand mismatch is severe enough, you'll have a heart attack or stroke and you may die. Since technological advancements allow us to have heart attacks and strokes and survive them, we don't usually die, but disease sets in, and our quality of life rapidly deteriorates. A recent study done in 2019 at the University of Melbourne in Australia revealed that our once life-saving measures for heart attacks are no longer working and we're seeing an increase of death from heart attacks despite taking extraordinary measures in treating them. This is also likely contributing to our decreasing life expectancy.

I learned a valuable lesson incorporating TCM into my practice. *The human body is self-aware and constantly communicating with its environment, both inside and outside the body, to assure survival and does so in ways that are ingenious, but not always obvious on the surface.* In today's unprecedented environment full of stressors, the body is constantly calculating how to maintain balance under these circumstances as nutrient and hormone levels decline. All this typically remains invisible in blood work and diagnostic/screening testing. Without the use of TCM, it's very difficult to see what's happening under the radar to correct them before diseases set in. Energy-based medicine has a central role in wellness and disease prevention because it provides the ability to see beneath the surface and treat the underlying causes of symptoms and correct them before they progress to the stage of disease. True prevention.

When Self-Correcting Forces Fail

Mainstream science has discovered fairly well-understood mechanisms for self-correction which can be found in the fields of epigenetics and genetics. DNA repair or repair of damaged genes occurs in all cells and involves up to 130 genes involved in reactions termed "DNA-damage response" or DDR. These are well-established and known mechanisms whereby *damaged genes can be repaired spontaneously in the cells of the body*. This doesn't mean that inherited mutated genes that we get from mother and father can be repaired. What I'm discussing here are genes that were normal at conception, but got damaged by the imbalanced environment inside your cells. It's very clear and accepted that there are certain genes whose sole job is to repair these other damaged genes.

We also have excellent documentation over several decades regarding stem cells as the body's innate repair mechanisms. These cells' functions are to go to areas throughout the body that send distress signals in order to replace those damaged or old cells. Stem cells generally become whatever cell surrounds them once they get to their destination. For example, if you place them in the liver, they become liver cells known as hepatocytes. If you place them in the heart, they become heart cells known as cardiomyocytes. They're signaled to where they're needed by the immune system producing inflammatory markers in response to damaged cells that require replacement.

If we have well-documented spontaneous repair mechanisms, why don't these mechanisms work and why do we still get diseases? In the next chapter, I'll discuss a very commonly used but equally misunderstood term: stress. We'll explore what stress really is and why and how it creates imbalance in the body's systems eventually breaking them.

CHAPTER FIVE

STRESS AND SELF-CORRECTING FORCES

But I Feel Fine. I'm Not Stressed

Everyone alive is familiar with stress. It's part of human life. We're currently reporting unprecedented stress here in the U.S. As stress goes on relentlessly for months or even years, the brain kicks in and helps keep the peace by normalizing the situation. If you actually perceive a significant amount of stress, your body will overreact and cause even more problems, but if you perceive situations as normal, your body's response is not so exaggerated. Under fight-or-flight, your blood pressure goes up, your heart starts to pound, you feel nervous and jumpy. If you assess the situation and see that there is no direct threat to your life, you can "talk" yourself down. What's wrong with that? That sounds pretty good, doesn't it?

What Is Stress Really?

While talking yourself down may be a good acute response to stressful situations, over time on a *cellular* level, your body ends up with a lot of balls to keep in the air as a result of chronic stress, and this requires more and more *energy*. Where does this energy come from? This energy comes from the foods you eat in the form of vitamins, minerals, antioxidants, proteins, fats, and carbohydrates. These nutrients mix with the oxygen you breathe to make energy. This energy is easily devoured by stress.

Stress You Can Feel and "Stealth" Stress

Stress in technical terms is anything — yes, *anything* — that causes imbalance in the body. What does that mean? Stress can be mental, such as a demanding boss in an understaffed office. You can feel the stress. You're on pins and needles. When you wake up in the morning, you're not so enthusiastic about going to work. You may have a feeling of dread at the thought or experience palpitations and mind racing. You may get very nervous and feel tired. This is an example of "*we become what we think*."

Stress can be physical, such as working 12-hour workdays, being sick with a cold or a chronic disease like diabetes, suffering from chronic pain, or having a prolonged cough that keeps you up at night. Having aches and pains that limit your movement or concentration and interrupt your sleep can be a physical stress. You can obviously feel this stress. Your brain chimes in and says, "Suck it up! You know you need this job. Get over it and get out of bed."

Then there is the stress you don't feel, stress that's not so obvious. I call this "*stealth*" or hidden stress. Stealth stress is the toxins in your environment, pesticides and synthetic ingredients in your foods such as food coloring or pesticides, unnatural products that get in through your skin such as lotions, or things that get inhaled such as aerosols. Why is this stressful?

When You Push Nature To Its Limits

Bodies have built-in mechanisms for detoxification and removal of waste, but remember that the human body evolved *into an environment suited for it*. We're built for the natural things that our bodies will encounter during an average lifespan. When it's exposed to unnatural products and chemicals, the body has to finagle a way to repackage these chemicals into a form that it can eliminate. Otherwise, these chemicals or toxins just keep recirculating in the body over and over leading to damage, disease, and even death. Our bodies are capable of repackaging and eliminating a lot, but they do have their limits.

Organisms have built-in mechanisms to evolve – another survival mechanism nature thought of in its perfection. For example, the Peppered moth evolved from the color white to gray/black in response to pollution in England, so it can remain camouflaged from its predators. If the moth wasn't capable of making this swift evolutionary change, it would be extinct. Moths have this survival mechanism so *why can't the human body do this*?

A moth lives anywhere from a few days up to one year, depending on the species. One moth can lay over 600 eggs at a time. The human lifespan, on the other hand, is quite long, and the female of our species can only reproduce one to two babies at a time from puberty until her thirties. Evolution takes many spans of reproduction to change genetic information that results in successful survival of a species. For humans, it takes thousands or even millions of years to change our genetic information. Our DNA or genetic code has remained exactly the same since we appeared on the planet 200,000 years ago! For the moth, it takes only a few years to change its genetic code, so the moth has a distinct advantage that we don't have.

Drastic Man-Made Environmental Changes

In the past century alone, mankind has drastically changed the environment with pesticides, genetically-modified foods, household chemicals, synthetic hormones that include birth control pills, synthetic pharmaceutical drugs, and much more. There are currently 80,000 man-made chemicals in our environment and we know very little about 99% of them in terms of their safety and their impact on the environment because we've only studied about 2,000 of them so far. It's a safe bet that most aren't doing the environment or our bodies any favors. Understanding this fact can be tricky because when we look at our sky, it still looks blue; when we look at our water, it still looks clear; and when we look at our soil, it looks the same as it always has. However, if we look *microscopically* at the sky, water and soil, we see the contamination that has occurred over the past century or two. What's important to know about this contamination of our environment is that the synthetic nature of these substances has created significant challenges for the body to rid itself of this toxic load. It's always critical to remember that the body is equipped to deal with *natural* things that were present in the environment when humans appeared 200,000 years ago - it's poorly equipped to deal with the synthetic and toxic chemicals to which it's exposed today. Pesticides alone are responsible for one million deaths worldwide every year.

The average American is exposed to 200 known cancer-causing synthetic toxins daily to say nothing about the other 78,000 toxins whose carcinogenicity we haven't yet investigated. It's been shown in studies that even babies are exposed to these toxins through the umbilical cord before they're even born, and this may be a critical link to the explosion of autism and childhood cancer rates of the past two decades.

The body is brilliant and prepared for stress, but when there are multiple toxins in addition to mental and physical stressors day in and day out, year after year, eventually it can't keep all those balls in the air, and trouble starts. Stress is an unsustainable strain on the body.

Man-Made Gender Role Changes

I may ruffle some feathers with this one, but stay with me. Women are outnumbering men in the workforce as part of the push for a dual-income family to handle the escalating costs of living caused by the industrial and technological revolutions, so we entered the workforce in droves starting in the 1970s.

Some are doctors like me, lawyers, engineers, military personnel, law enforcement personnel, business executives, clerical professionals, teachers, etc. We do it all, and we do it well! *What has this done to us in terms of stress, however*? These side effects are not so obvious until you look under the surface. According to TCM, stress consumes blood and this is significant for women as we'll see next.

Another premise of TCM is that "women are of *blood* and men are of *qi*" (vital energy). What does this mean? Women use blood for their natural roles as nurturers. They get pregnant, and this requires blood to feed the baby. Blood production increases by 50% during a pregnancy. They breastfeed their children. Breast milk is made of blood. If they aren't either pregnant or breastfeeding, they menstruate monthly until menopause. This also consumes blood. According to traditional Chinese medicine, women are of blood and when you think about it, it makes sense.

Men, on the other hand, are traditionally the hunter-gatherers, and they are made of *qi* (pronounced chee) or vital energy. Men and women both have qi and blood, so relatively speaking women use more of their blood, and men use more of their qi or vital energy. Therefore, it makes sense that men are of qi. Men don't get pregnant, breastfeed or menstruate so they don't require blood in their natural roles as hunter-gatherers.

As women entered the workforce, they *became hunter-gatherers as well as nurturers* and started using large amounts of qi (vital energy) and blood. The problem is that men cannot take over women's evolutionary role of pregnancy and breastfeeding, so we've kept these roles in addition to our new roles as hunter-gatherers.

To make matters worse, monthly menstruation also uses a lot of blood. If we think about menstruation throughout history, women actually didn't menstruate very much throughout their reproductive years in the remote past. Women menstruated at the onset of puberty or menarche, and frequently got pregnant shortly thereafter. There is no menstruation during pregnancy. After a woman gave birth, the primary mechanism to feed her baby was breastfeeding around the clock. Women who consistently breastfeed around the clock don't menstruate or get pregnant. Women would often breastfeed for several years to nourish their babies. Once they stopped breastfeeding, their menstruation would resume and they'd get pregnant again. And around and around this went until menopause, if they lived long enough to experience menopause. Women of the remote past didn't menstruate nearly as much as modern women, so modern women use and lose a lot more blood than women of the past, which sets us up for problems. Again, we manage this really well on the surface, but if we add to those circumstances the toxins and stress that we encounter daily as we move through life, that spells trouble for us if we're not careful.

Another not-so-obvious role change is how children are raised. In the distant past, children were raised with other men and women in a village. This provided protection from predators and also allowed a significant group of women to band together to care for their young, which made it easier in certain ways. Today, children are raised in relative isolation. A mother or father may rush them to daycare on the way to work, or raise them alone in the home. Although men have helped women more and more, this isn't enough. I've always believed that stay-at-home moms work harder than women in the workforce because there are labor laws in the workforce that aren't present in the American home. Women work tirelessly at home, often without breaks. This spells trouble long-term. Welch's juice company conducted a survey of 2,000 moms in 2016 which showed that the average mom works an average of 14 hours a day or 98 hours a week including weekends, which is the equivalent of 2.5 full-time jobs!!

Given what we know about stress consuming blood, we can now see how it manifest in terms of disease. Women are twice as likely as men to suffer from depression. According to the National Institutes of Health (NIH), a startling 78% of autoimmune disorders, such as rheumatoid arthritis and systemic lupus, occur in women!

The *basis for this is well known in traditional Chinese medicine*, yet it's not easily understood in conventional medicine. In TCM the patterns of disharmony responsible for conditions and symptoms such as depression and autoimmune disorders have well-described patterns of disharmony and can be addressed from their root causes. Many of them have to do with overworking, emotions, and stress, which clearly impact women differently than men as we just discussed. Stress directly impacts the blood and can consume blood or cause it to stagnate resulting in poor circulation; this affects women more than men because of their utilization of blood and explains why women are more prone to these conditions.

In the next chapter, I'll discuss a particular type of psychological stress caused by poorly processed emotions driven by fear-based thinking.

CHAPTER SIX

EMOTIONS AND DISEASE

Emotions Are Energy In Motion

$E= mc^2$. Albert Einstein showed us that energy becomes matter; therefore, so do emotions since emotions are a type of energy. Science is proving what we already knew, but for what it's worth, we now have evidence that we create our perception of reality through our thoughts. Emotions are triggered by thoughts and therefore create a perception of how we see the world and ourselves in it. Thoughts are not just things, they become our reality. We become what we think regardless of whether these thoughts are conscious or *subconscious*.

How we process emotions and thoughts create chemical reactions in the body that can lead to wellness or disease. The choice, believe it or not, is yours. Your cells are directed by your feelings and thoughts, which translate into body instructions on a biochemical level: hormones, vitamins, minerals, antioxidants, and oxygen, each playing its role to express gene function and body function 24 hours a day.

How Negative Emotions Breed Disease

Does that mean that we are responsible for our diseases? Technically the answer to this question is yes; however, if you can "catch" or become aware of your thoughts as they come out of your subconscious mind, you can transform them into positive thoughts to positively impact your health. If you live your life unaware, your subconscious mind runs it for you, and negative thoughts arise where positive thoughts are not cultivated. *Negative emotions are a special form of stress*, which is not often recognized. If we suppress our emotions and try to be positive, this also represents a stress. While we may believe that we're not responsible for our diseases, if we look deeply at this question, we begin to see that we are. Again, it may be on a subconscious level and you may not even be aware that you're driving the process. Those who can become aware of this reality can begin to consciously change their thinking and heal. Genuinely positive emotions are healing and help reduce the impact of stress.

Nature abhors a vacuum. Mind your thoughts and feelings or your subconscious will fill in the blanks with negative ones. This is much like tending to a garden. If we don't tend to our garden, weeds grow instead of the beautiful flowers, vegetables, or fruits that we've planted. This is a well-known concept in Eastern philosophies but not well known in Western societies. It is, however, a universal law.

We also see this in science, as we know that all things in the third dimension naturally tend toward disorder if they're not purposefully organized. This is called the Second Law of Thermodynamics in physics. This law, discovered around 1850, revealed the natural tendency of any isolated system to degenerate into a more disordered state. Simply put, all things in the third dimension of reality have a tendency to get messier and messier unless energy is put back into the system to reorganize it. Our bodies are no different. This is why we have to eat properly, learn proper breathing techniques, and still the mind to properly "feed" the body to keep it from falling apart.

While these strategies sound simplistic, these are the secrets to wellness as we'll discuss. Einstein's equation $E = mc^2$ was initially scoffed at due to its incredible simplicity, but it turned out to be a game-changer in modern physics giving birth to modern space travel, satellite and cell phone technology, and more. Don't underestimate simplicity - it's the language of the universe! There is mounting evidence that the entire universe is connected, not just as it exists here in the third dimension, but across multiple dimensions outside of space and time. I mention dimensions because we are rapidly finding out that there are multiple dimensions at work around our planet, and the laws differ for each of them. Ancient texts report that there are 12 dimensions around the earth. Scientists have discovered 11 of them so far and astonishingly, there's emerging evidence as published by the Blue Brain Project out of Geneva, Switzerland, that the mouse brain is capable of "thinking" in all 11 of these dimensions. Since the mouse and human are so similar, it's a huge step in understanding the human brain and gaining an understanding that learning to care for our mind, body and spirit allows us to exist across dimensions and to truly be whole.

When I wrote my first book *The Tao of Integrative Medicine*, published in 2016, I was aware of The HeartMath® Institute in California, but what I've subsequently learned of their ground-breaking research is fascinating. In 1991, Dr. Andrew Armour of the University of Montreal discovered a complex set of 40,000 neurons in the heart that he coined the *"heart-brain."* These neurons work on multiple levels and were discovered to have *independent* complex processing and *memory* capabilities. What this meant is that the heart-brain could make decisions regarding heart function *independent of the central nervous system.* In other words, the brain in your heart makes decisions independent of the brain in your head!

The heart-brain was also connected to the head-brain on a different level, meaning that the emotions and rhythms felt in the heart communicated with the head-brain which then affected the *entire body*, not just the heart, through transmission via the nervous system. In fact, there are many more nerves that travel from the heart-brain to the head-brain than the other way around!

This was completely counter to what we knew about the heart for centuries in modern medicine, BUT *completely in line with what ancient traditions and energy-based systems of medicine teach us.* According to traditional Chinese medicine, the heart houses the mind! The Institute of HeartMath® in California has done some ground-breaking research over the past 20-30 years related to emotions, thoughts and disease. They show through decades of research that heart rate *variability* provides a consistent measure of stress and emotions. Negative emotions felt in the heart region cause disorder in heart rate variability, which impacts the autonomic (subconscious) nervous system causing adverse reactions throughout the body. This is called *non-coherence*.

Positive emotions felt in the heart region lead to order, balance, and harmony in our heart rate variability, which impacts the autonomic nervous system causing balance and harmony in the body. This is called *coherence*. **Coherence occurs when we synchronize or harmonize the "heart-brain" with the "head-brain" so that both work optimally for the balance of our body and mind.**

A study published in the April-June, 1998 issue of *Integrative Physiological and Behavioral Science* showed a remarkable 100% increase of DHEA (the "anti-aging" hormone made by the adrenal glands) and a 23% reduction of cortisol (the chronic stress hormone also made by the adrenal glands) with an emotional self-management program consisting of specific *simple* steps that lead to positive emotions and lessen negative thought loops. We can measure autonomic nervous system tracings by measuring heart rate variability through biofeedback technology. There are specific patterns that are seen with what's called coherence vs non-coherence. When we're in coherence we're "in sync" and levels of cortisol are low and DHEA increases for an anti-aging effect. Blood pressure and heart rate are also lower when we're in coherence. Being in coherence correlates with the portion of the autonomic nervous system called the parasympathetic nervous system. This is the "calming" portion of the nervous system which is activated by positive emotions of joy, calm, gratitude, and love. This is supposed to be our natural state of being. With practice, we can form a positive feedback loop, in other words, train the body to stay on this wavelength, which is actually our default state of being that we've lost touch with. See figure 3.

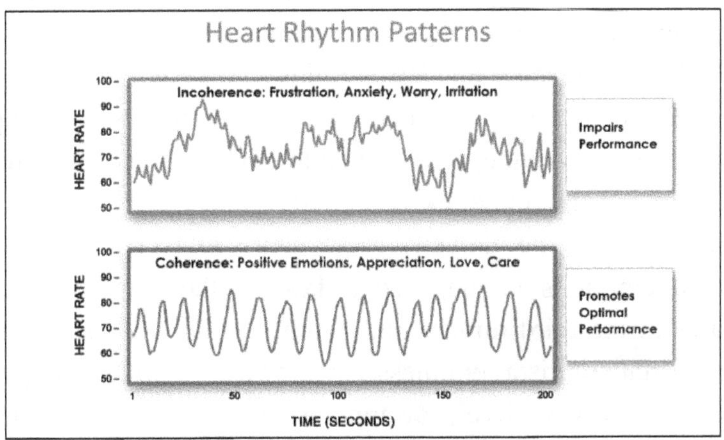

Figure 3: Heart Rhythm Patterns – incoherent heart variability patterns (in red) versus coherent heart variability patterns (in blue). Achieving coherence promotes wellbeing and optimal performance whereas incoherence or non-coherence promotes anxiety and can breed disease. Credit: HeartMath®.org

---

The sympathetic nervous system is the stress "fight-or-flight" portion of the autonomic nervous system which increases cortisol and lowers DHEA. The sympathetic nervous system also increases blood pressure and heart rate. We experience this during times of stress and fight-or-flight responses. *This isn't supposed to be our default state, but our modern stressful lifestyles have "trained" us to stay on this wavelength instead of our default state.* When chronically active, these destructive sets of chemical reactions lead to imbalance, disease and even death.

How Negative Emotions Gain Control

Negative emotions are a kind of place-holder if positive thoughts aren't there. This is a universal law that operates in the third dimension just like the law of gravity. Universal laws just are. You don't have to believe in them because they exist whether you do or not. If we don't have a healthy respect for universal laws, we pay the consequences. We teach our children not to jump out of windows like Superman because we know that even if that child believes she or he can fly, the third dimensional qualities of gravity will quickly correct those misperceptions. The universal law that's at work in the case of negative emotions is the second law of thermodynamics, which operates in the third dimension, which says that a system will tend toward a state of disorder unless you actively pump the energy in it to keep it orderly. If we live unaware, the subconscious fills in the blanks and things get messy just like the garden that was ignored and is now full of weeds. *As children, we internalize every emotion and every experience*. Whether we remember an event or not, we remember the flavor of the experience, and this creates pathways in the head-brain if we don't learn at an early age how to process emotions and don't see this processing demonstrated by our parents and caretakers.

The head-brain is very plastic, and loops are formed throughout childhood until about the age of 25 when they become more or less hardwired if we're not careful. They tend to be so ingrained that they're almost permanent, so the brain keeps looping the same stories over and over again. This forms a loop of unconscious stress if our early experiences were stressful. Considering that unborn children are exposed to up to 180 known dangerous toxins which cause immediate stress, this is a key factor to keep in awareness.

This hardwiring starts when we're kids. Every experience with every person, place, or thing since childhood is programmed into our brains. We tend to function from past experiences before we act because our brains cannot process the 15,000,000 bits of data bombarding us every second. The extra data we can't process in the moment goes to the subconscious mind. It's our subconscious mind that reminds us that the hot stove hurts, so we remember this before we decide not to touch it. This is of course a very important function for survival, but *if we don't learn to distinguish what's important from our past from what's just based in fear for its own sake, trouble starts.* For example, if we hear as children that "money doesn't grow on trees" or "we can't afford that," the fear that this causes subconsciously and the thoughts they evoke remain with us throughout our lives and may cause financial difficulties if we're not consciously aware of the feelings and thoughts hanging out in our subconscious and work to change them. Our external experiences and the emotions they evoke "train" us to keep thinking along those familiar lines. We continue to have similar experiences with different people and circumstances, but it's the same story over and over because these stories are hardwired since childhood and recalled throughout our lives.

A monumental study done in England followed thousands of children starting in 1958 until they reached age 45. Their teachers were asked to answer a 146-question assessment of these children at ages seven, 11, and 16. At age 45 they were assessed, looking for indicators of chronic disease as this was the endpoint of the study. Chronic diseases were noted to be more common in kids exposed to stress early in their lives even if the stress didn't persist through adulthood. In other words, the children who experienced childhood stress were significantly more likely to have chronic diseases in adulthood. Even if these children didn't have stress during adulthood, they had a significant risk of chronic diseases. This study was published by the *Journal of the American College of Cardiology* in 2015. Childhood experiences can have life-long impacts unless we're aware and consciously choose to change our thought patterns.

Reversing the Negativity

In Chinese medical theory, which is over 4,000 years old, there is a premise that the "heart houses the mind." In 1991, The Institute of HeartMath® discovered 40,000 "brain" cells in the human heart, essentially proving this Chinese medical premise to be true. The Institute of HeartMath® also discovered a neural network between the heart brain and head brain, and there were many more neural connections going *from the heart to the head brain* than from the head brain to the heart.

There is also a very powerful electromagnetic field emanating from the heart which is 100X more powerful than any other fields in our bodies. Scientifically we don't know how far it extends because this field maxed out the machines designed to measure it. They estimated that this electromagnetic field goes out at least 8-11 feet.

Metaphysically or spiritually it's understood that this electromagnetic field is infinite. These heart-brain cells aren't influenced by the ego, like our head-brain is. Through the use of the heart, communication is not filtered by the ego, so we circumvent the fear, apprehension, and past memories that trigger fear-based thinking. This electromagnetic field that emanates from the heart is not bound by space and time if it is indeed infinite. There's significant evidence that particles or photons are instantaneously in communication no matter how far apart they are. They communicate outside of space and time. The heart-brain appears to operate based on this principle. In fact, experienced meditators who are in high coherence can accurately predict events before they happen. There is significant evidence to suggest that the physical heart is connected to a field that is not limited to space and time as we currently understand it. The heart receives and processes information about an event BEFORE the event takes place. There's also evidence that this happens on a global scale. The study conducted at Princeton University is likely the most famous of these experiments. I'll discuss this study in chapter 12.

Ultimately, we need to *use both our heart-brain and head-brain in harmony*. Meditation and proper breathing techniques allow the harmonization of the heart and head-brains, so they work optimally with each other. When we allow the head-brain to bleed into thoughts it's not supposed to have and involve the ego, we get lost. When we begin to use our head-brain to try to conform to what others think, we get lost quickly. The reason is that we're focusing our thoughts in the wrong place! Our head-brain is for logical thinking such as directions to get somewhere, how to add 2 + 2 to equal 4; how to bake a cake, or plant a garden. Head-brain is also for something even more important: survival. It reminds us that fire is hot or detects that predators are nearby. When we begin to ask our head-brain if we're being judged or if we've done something shameful or embarrassing, we're off on a tangent that the head-brain cannot process. Head-brain then goes into survival mode and begins to create stories and possibilities that revolve around *past* subconscious or conscious experiences which are ego- and fear-based thinking. This triggers what feels like a never-ending bombardment of thoughts, which sets up more fear-based thinking in a negative loop. We've all caught ourselves day dreaming with doomsday scenarios over what ended up being minor situations.

When we begin to distinguish what the heart-brain is responsible for and what the head brain is responsible for, we can merge them and allow harmonization. When we ask our heart-brain a question it answers from a position of our higher selves where there is no fear, no judgment, and no story. There is only Truth. It's critical to begin with the outcome as though it's already done! We're physical linear beings and *also* quantum, infinite beings as we'll discuss later when we review how the latest scientific research is verifying ancient traditions. We're much more than what meets the eye! The field of quantum physics is driving this point home!

Thankfully, our head-brain is much more plastic than previously thought, so we can change this hardwiring by synchronizing with the heart's electromagnetic field. To begin to reverse the broken records in our subconscious minds, we have to first notice that they exist in the first place. My five Cs of change are as follows:

1. The first step is becoming ***conscious*** that you have a problem with negative emotions and thoughts.
2. The second step is making a ***commitment*** to capture these thoughts as they arise and
3. ***choose*** to see them differently.
4. Then consistently ***cultivate*** this behavioral change by stilling the mind with meditation and specific breathing techniques.

5. Be ***consistent*** in practicing these principles for the rest of your life. You'll slip occasionally, but if you practice with these 5 Cs in mind, you'll get back up and keep doing your work with great results!

Meditation has been proven to change brain patterns and rewire the brain, both physically and mentally. This helps explain why meditation has been shown to be a great stress reliever. It quiets the brain over time and allows heart-based thinking to predominate rather than fear-based or head-brain thinking. Functional MRI studies have been done in novice meditators to prove this. The trick is you have to keep doing it, or the work gets undone — just like you have to keep tending to that garden or the weeds take over. As our practice in meditation matures, we can endeavor to be in meditation as we move through our day. In other words, we choose to keep the mind still all day as we move through the various experiences of life such as waking up, preparing for the day, greeting our family and friends, participating in everyday activities. In spiritual speak, this relates to "being *in* the world, yet not *of* the world."

The Institute of HeartMath® has also studied shorter heart-based breathing techniques lasting only 3 minutes, whose effects have been shown to last up to 6 hours. This allows a "recycling" of stillness throughout the day if repeated 3 times daily. Although this sounds too simple to be true, always remember that *simplicity is the language of the Universe*!

These methods allow for an awareness to develop over time. Instantaneous change is not usually possible, so patience with yourself as you develop these practices is critical. Self-love and acceptance are the keys to making permanent changes! While the circumstances of life may continue, it's *how you process and choose to react, or not react, that makes all the difference*. This doesn't mean that we become complacent like sitting ducks and accept whatever's happening. It means that we become aware of what is and choose not to make a story out of it. We choose to simply be aware *and at the same time*, begin to develop a different story that has the desired end in mind as though it were already done! The Institute of HeartMath® stresses that the link to your emotions is critical. You can't stuff them, ignore them, or otherwise pretend they're not there. You must choose to experience them and allow them to pass naturally. This may require the assistance of a therapist or counselor and may not be something everyone can do alone.

Ultimately however, we must all choose to experience and know that emotions, symptoms, and diseases *are not* who we are. *They are experiences we have.* Learning to dis-identify with an emotion or disease is critical to letting it go. This is not the same as stuffing or suppressing an emotion or experience of disease. It's critical to understand the difference. When you stuff or suppress an emotion, you create a loop in your subconscious that holds on to this negative emotion and keeps bringing it back with future experiences. This is how the head-brain works. The subconscious mind and its memories are processed in the head-brain and can be found in all of our cells. There's emerging scientific data that cells retain memory as previously discussed. This leads to physical changes in the body that are destructive because the emotional energy was retained in the body. This is how a symptom or disease takes hold. To "undo" a symptom or disease, you reverse-engineer the experience of emotion by letting it pass through the body and not get stuck inside the body's subconscious head-brain and cells.

When you allow yourself to feel the emotion and process it in a safe environment, whether with a therapist, counselor or alone, you involve the heart-brain which can then properly synchronize and release the emotion, so it doesn't get stuck in your subconscious. Again, remember that this process isn't instantaneous and other experiences will come along and require the same approach. It's a long-term practice in mastery.

Nature abhors a vacuum. Never let up, or you'll go backwards. Maintaining the awareness of heart-centered thinking allows the head-brain and fear-based thinking to subside. It creates space to allow for more positive emotions. Harmonizing the heart and the head-brain allows us to process information with minimal stress and regain and maintain health and wellness over time. *Always remember that you are in full control of your experience through the processing of your emotions, whether the experience is perceived as good or bad.*

As emotions are known to be "energy in motion," you, as the observer of your emotions, are critical in determining what will happen *within you and manifest in your world* as a result of the experience of the emotion! In other words, how we process our emotions will determine how our body responds to the experience of the emotion. Energy should keep moving, not get stuck. When we suppress emotions, we slow them down and they get stuck in our subconscious minds and in our cells. When we allow them to pass through us, we keep them moving, which allows for positive emotions to flow through. This is a very liberating realization as we begin to really know and understand that we are, in fact, in full control of our total experience including our health, wholeness and wellness.

Chinese medicine has a lot to say about emotions or energy in motion since it's an energy-based system of medicine. In fact, according to TCM, the main ***internal*** causes of disease are emotions! There are 7 emotions which cause disease according to TCM. They are:

- Anger
- Joy (excessive joy as in craving or addiction)
- Sadness
- Worry
- Pensiveness (brooding or rumination)
- Fear (both sudden and chronic)
- Shock

According to TCM theory, all emotions have effects on qi or vital energy, and can lead to disease when either prolonged or intense.

- *Anger* makes qi (vital energy) rise and affects the **liver** and **gallbladder** directly.
- *Joy* slows down qi and affects the **heart** and **small intestine** directly.
- *Sadness* depletes qi and affects the **lung** and **large intestine** directly.
- *Worry* stagnates or knots qi and affects the **spleen** and **stomach** (related to the gastrointestinal system) directly.
- *Pensiveness* also knots qi and also affects the **spleen** and **stomach** directly.
- *Fear* makes qi descend and affects the **kidneys** and **bladder** directly.
- *Shock* scatters qi and also affects the **kidneys** and **bladder** directly.

All prolonged or intense emotions affect the heart either directly or indirectly because the *heart houses the Mind* according to TCM theory. An imbalance of an internal organ can also cause emotional imbalances according to TCM. The organs and emotions are resonant and interdependent. This resonance allows us to heal emotional trauma using acupuncture, herbs, and sound therapy. The link between all emotions and the heart also explains the global coherence phenomenon well, which we'll discuss more in chapter 12.

The 6 Healing Sounds in TCM are a form of qi gong, which is a form of moving meditation and breathing. Qi gong is actually a very powerful form of medicine and self-healing practiced in China for thousands of years. It helps compliment the healing techniques practiced in TCM clinics and gives the patient the power to continue the healing practice at home. Combining qi gong with sound therapy has also been practiced in China for thousands of years. The theory of the 6 healing sounds states that each organ corresponds to a sound that if practiced in combination with qi gong techniques, allows each organ to remove stale qi or emotions and replace the stale qi with fresh qi, and the negative emotions with positive emotions.

The 6 Healing Sounds of TCM are based on the resonant sounds of the major organs of TCM and are as follows:

- Lung/Large Intestine sound: "Sssssss"
- Kidney/Bladder sound: "Chooooo"
- Liver/Gallbladder sound: "Shhhhhh"
- Heart/Small Intestine sound: "Hawwww"
- Spleen/Stomach sound: "Heeeeeee"

For more detailed information on performing the 6 Healing Sounds, I invite you to read *Chi Nei Tsang* by Mantak Chia.

Although ancient Chinese physicians didn't perform clinical studies as we know them today, this practice has survived thousands of years and the field of vibroacoustics or sound therapy is evolving today with sound clinical research to back its use. A study released in the journal *Pain Research and Management* in 2015 showed vibroacoustic therapy to be effective for relieving the pain associated with fibromyalgia. Another study completed in 2009 in the journal *NeuroRehabilitation* showed improvement in symptoms of Parkinson's disease. A study released in 2018 in the *Journal of Biology and Medical Research* showed significant improvement of postoperative pain and speedier recovery from knee surgery.

A more recent medical study published in the journal *Cell* in March 2019 by scientists at the Massachusetts Institute of Technology, showed that Alzheimer's dementia plaques in mice could be dissolved by light and sound therapies. It will take quite some time for our modern research to catch up to the thousands of years of clinical practice in the field of TCM, but in my experience, TCM is always the right path to pursue for symptoms and conditions that are not immediately life-threatening. I'll discuss this amazing energy-based system of medicine next.

CHAPTER SEVEN

TRADITIONAL CHINESE MEDICINE

How Did They Know?

Eastern philosophies have always fascinated me. How did they know? As a child, I often wondered how a seed knew which way to grow when it was planted in the ground. Why didn't it grow into the ground instead of moving toward the surface?

I eventually concluded that it must be connected somehow to the whole and simply knows which way to grow. After all, a plant doesn't have an ego constantly clamoring in its head telling it which way to go and how to get there. It just knows.

Chinese medicine, which is over 4,000 years old, is based on what is now called quantum physics: that spooky, weird science that no one can really understand today, but it's used in many different ways most people aren't aware of. The use of cell phone technology, space travel, and more is based in quantum physics. In fact, many body functions like our sense of smell, for example, are now being recognized as being based in quantum physics. We are, in fact, quantum beings.

Modern science in the West only began to discover the principles of quantum physics a little over 100 years ago. Ancient Chinese physicians used these principles over 4,000 years ago!

Neils Bohr, one of the fathers of quantum physics in the West, once said, “If quantum mechanics hasn’t profoundly shocked you, you haven’t understood it yet.” But it exists and is used to power cell phones, send people to the moon, launch satellites, and it works consistently every time. Why? It’s based on universal laws, that’s why. Universal laws aren’t sneaky or tricky. Universal laws don’t change regardless of what’s going on. Gravity and the laws of thermodynamics are good examples of universal laws operational in the third dimension. If you observe universal laws carefully, they teach you a lot about yourself and your role in the universe as a spiritual being having a human experience of yourself in this dimension!

As humans, we are part of the whole, and we cannot be separated from the whole. Considering what humanity has done to its environment in the past hundred years, this is a critical piece of information to know. Basically, what we do to the environment we do to ourselves!

If we follow this principle, it also means that **every dysfunction or disease is related to the whole and cannot be treated in an isolated fashion.** TCM emphasizes that every small part of the body reflects the whole and bases its evaluations on this premise.

In 1905 an American biologist, Edwin Grant Conklin, made a startling observation while studying small marine animals called tunicates which led to the biological proof that every small part of the body does, in fact, reflect the whole. According to the article in *Discover Magazine* the contents of the tunicate mother egg, Conklin discovered, weren’t uniform. Different parts of it were differently colored. When the mother egg began to divide, the new daughter cells, naturally enough, took their cellular matter from the part of the egg from which they'd arisen. What surprised Conklin, however, was that the daughter cells that came from different-colored areas of the mother egg became different types of tissues in the daughter eggs. The yellow stuff in the mother egg produced muscle cells in the daughter eggs, and the grayish stuff that split from the mother egg became the cells that formed the gut in the daughter tunicates. Some substance in each part of the mother egg was acting to shunt each daughter cell down a different developmental path to create different types of tissues in the offspring. Later experiments confirmed that different parts of the mother egg can indeed dictate the fate of their daughter cells by using proteins to activate (or deactivate) the relevant developmental genes.

This observation is startling because the *genetic code that determines this is very consistent for many different species from flies to humans*! Human cells divide in a similar way, and the part of the human mother egg from which the daughter cell comes determines what type of cell it will become; **every small part reflects the whole**! For example, cells that come from the front part of the egg will become the head, and cells that come from the back of the same egg will become the feet. That one little egg from which we come has the whole body mapped out in it. Incredible!

Additional evidence of this premise can be found in the human genome itself. Thanks to modern scientific inquiry, we have proven that every single cell in the human body has the genetic code of the entire body in it. Cells seem to have a consciousness all their own and know that they are heart cells when they are part of the heart, for example, and not skin cells. This is based on the environment around the cell and also follows the principles of quantum physics. These principles are very aligned with traditional Chinese medicine theories since they are all based on this philosophy that we are now proving with science.

Although ancient Chinese physicians didn't have this technology, they came to the same conclusion and created an entire system of medicine based on this concept thousands of years ago.

The balance of energies between the part and the whole must be considered for effective understanding of how to treat a disease. Traditional Chinese medicine is based on the maintenance of balance between energies called *yin*, which in the body, is vital essence, and *yang*, which, in the body, is vital function.

Yin and *yang* are very complex, yet very elegant and simple concepts, and what I am expressing in this book doesn't even begin to address their true functions. A crude way of understanding *yin* is to see it as substance or matter. *Yang* is understood as a function and activity of that substance or matter, so the anatomy of the body is considered *yin*, and the function or physiology is considered *yang*.

Just as we cannot separate the body from its functions and maintain life, we cannot separate *yin* from *yang*, or we would cease to be alive. Everything in the universe has *yin* and *yang* qualities. The moon is considered to be *yin*, compared to the sun, which is considered *yang*. Night is considered *yin*, compared to day, which is considered *yang*.

***YIN* QUALITIES**	***YANG* QUALITIES**
Moon	Sun
Earth	Heavens
Female	Male
Negative Charge	Positive Charge
Cold	Hot
Night	Day

Yin and *yang* are only significant when they are related to each other. We know this as the concept of duality. We would not know what night is without the concept of day. We cannot understand the concept of cold without the concept of hot. Alone they wouldn't mean much.

We can approximate the meanings of *yin* and *yang* by isolating them, but they are only really understood when they are related to each other — kind of like people. Isolated we can do some things, but together we can do great things.

Yin and *yang* cannot be separated, or life would cease to exist. They are interrelated at all times. Even in the highest *yang* possible, there is *yin* and vice versa. At high noon, there is a tiny little seed of night, and that tiny little seed grows as your day continues until night takes over, and there is more *yin* than *yang*. Even at midnight, there is a tiny little seed of day that will grow into full day, so *yin* and *yang* are constantly interrelated in this way. This is demonstrated in the illustration of the *yin-yang* symbol in figure 4. There is a small circle in each symbol which represents that tiny seed.

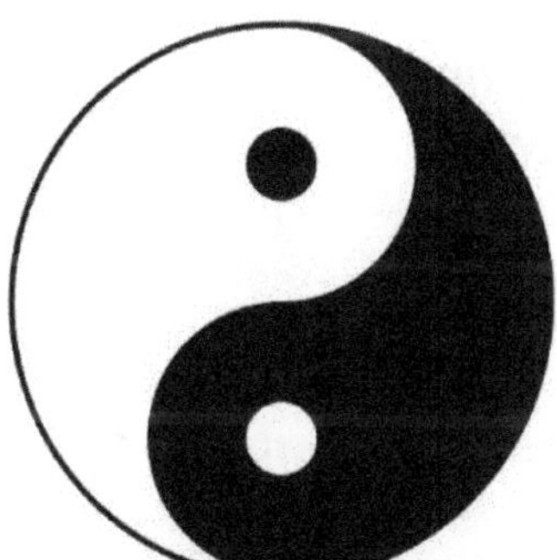

Figure 4: The yin-yang symbol is called taijitu and is a visual representation of the qualities of *yin* and *yang* energies of the universe. The illustration depicts two interlocking spirals with dots of the opposing color in the middle of each spiral. The black spiral represents *yin*, and the white spiral represents *yang*. The dots in the center represent the presence of a small amount of *yin* (black dot) in the highest *yang* and a small amount of *yang* (white dot) in the highest *yin*. The symbol also depicts how *yin* becomes *yang* and vice versa. The third quality depicted by the illustration is how *yin* supports *yang* and vice versa. The fourth quality depicted is how *yin* controls *yang* and vice versa. This visual representation helps us see how *yin* and *yang* are related in all parts of the universe.

In a nutshell, *yin* is relatively solid, earth, grounded, cold, low-vibrating, and quiet. *Yang*, on the other hand, is airy, light, heaven, hot, high-vibrating, and loud. Those are some qualities of *yin* and *yang*. They are somewhat opposite, but their relationship is way deeper than that.

Because they're somewhat opposite, they keep each other in check. They **support** each other, and they **become** each other. *Yin* can become *yang*, and *yang* can become *yin*. This is called inter-transformation. We understand these concepts as day becoming night and night becoming day. *Yin* **consumes** and **controls** *yang*, and *yang* **consumes** and **controls** *yin*. There is a balance maintained between these two energies that keep the peace.

The universe is self-maintaining and self-correcting. There is very little we have to do if we keep the harmony between ourselves and our environment. The earth spins around the sun, but there are unseen forces keeping the earth from spinning into the sun or too far away from it. This is *yin* and *yang* at work. The same concept is at work in the human body and every other entity in the universe. As above, so below. The body's self-correcting forces are *yin* and *yang* at work.

The Five Elements of TCM

The theory of the five elements originated about 3,000 years ago. According to the ancient Chinese text Shang Shu "The five elements are water, fire, wood, metal and earth. Water moistens downward, fire flares upwards, wood can be bent and straightened, metal can be molded and can harden, earth permits sowing, growing and reaping."

The five elements have very critical relationships to each other. One very important relationship is the **generation cycle** which states that wood generates fire, fire generates earth, earth generates metal,

metal generates water, and water generates wood, which starts the cycle anew.

Another cycle is the **controlling cycle** which states that fire controls metal, metal controls wood, wood controls earth, earth controls water, and water controls fire. We see examples of this in nature: a metal ax can chop wood, water can extinguish a fire, and the earth contains bodies of water.

The five elements have many more relationships outside of the scope of this book, but they explain natural phenomena extremely well and accurately, which provides the basis of its use in medicine. Each element also corresponds to certain organs of the human body as follows:

- Metal: Lung (yin) and Large Intestine (yang)
- Water: Kidney (yin) and Bladder (yang)
- Wood: Liver (yin) and Gallbladder (yang)
- Fire: Heart (yin) and Small Intestine (yang)
- Earth: Spleen (yin) and Stomach (yang)

How Traditional Chinese Medicine (TCM) Adds Value To Evaluation and Treatment of Disease

In the human body, certain organs have relatively *yin* qualities, and others have relatively *yang* qualities. For example, as stated previously the liver is a *yin* organ, and the gallbladder is a *yang* organ but only when related to each other. Within the liver there is *yin* and *yang*, and within the gallbladder there is also *yin* and *yang*. They are inseparable.

In the heart there is *yin* and *yang*. They are what keep your heart beating at a balanced pace. If there is an imbalance of *yin* and *yang* in the heart, you can have an abnormal heart rhythm or even have a heart attack. If there is insufficient *yin* — or calming energy — in the heart, the heart beats too fast. If there is not enough *yang*, or fire, in the heart, it beats too slowly.

Principles of traditional Chinese medicine are well beyond the scope of this book, but essentially, it's about balance between a person and his or her environment. When we are out of harmony for too long, we get sick.

In traditional Chinese medicine, through the use of what is called "the four examinations," symptoms or diseases can be evaluated, and the patterns of disharmony (or root causes of symptoms) can be determined without any testing.

The evaluation always takes the individual's environment into consideration. There is no such thing as "psychosomatic" in traditional Chinese medicine. In other words, we never think an illness is just in somebody's head because every symptom has a cause, and it's related in some way to the whole. They're absolutely inseparable.

In traditional Chinese medicine, placebo is important because the Mind controls wellness. We discount placebo in conventional medicine and see it as unimportant; however, the placebo effect is critically important because if we think a certain thought, it triggers distinct physiological changes, so placebo is critical. It's all considered because TCM sees the unseen connections between all things in the universe.

A study reported in the *New England Journal of Medicine* in 2002 revealed that arthroscopic knee surgery for arthritis was no better than placebo. Patients were "told" they had surgery after a small incision was made in their knee by the surgeon, but no surgery was performed. Other patients had actual knee surgery. According to the study: "At no point did either of the intervention groups report less pain or better function than the placebo group." In other words, the people that never had surgery but thought they did, reported improvement at the same rate as those who had actual surgery. We become what we think!

Thoughts leading to chemical reactions in the body are proven in science, so placebo is just as important as anything else that helps someone be well. In the 1970s, a concept called "downward causation" was discovered by modern science. This is the idea that higher systems influence lower systems based on a joint interaction with the environment. An example is that mental events cause physical events: the placebo effect as we just discussed! These events cannot take place without the environment. Just as positive thoughts of being told you've had knee surgery to eliminate your knee pain cause positive chemical reactions in the body to eliminate pain, it's also very clear now that negative thoughts cause destructive chemical reactions in the body via complex mechanisms involving the nervous system.

This concept of downward causation has been known for thousands of years in Eastern philosophies: "We become what we think." The field of quantum physics is showing that thoughts are now known to be a form of energy, and this form of energy can become matter because $E = mc^2$. In other words, thoughts become things! They say you are what you eat. An even more important saying is you become what you think.

The real value of traditional Chinese medicine is how it *explains the cause* of symptoms and does more than diagnose a condition. It actually tells you *why* you have a condition and *how* you can correct it. This is unheard of in our conventional system of medicine.

In allopathic medicine, we diagnose then treat diseases by blocking expression of the symptom, which does absolutely nothing to cure the condition. It saves lives when the symptom is life-threatening, but it doesn't help prevent another occurrence or prevent the condition from spiraling into yet another condition.

Another startling difference between TCM and allopathic medicine that has huge implications is how we treat infections. In allopathic medicine, we sometimes allow infections to run their course and assume that the immune system will deal with the intruder, or we treat with antibiotics.

In life-threatening infection, antibiotics are critical for saving lives; however, in infections that are not serious, antibiotics simply weaken the immune system further, leaving us prey to other infections. The fact that antibiotics weaken immunity is not well accepted in allopathic medicine, but can easily be explained by the destabilization of the microbiome in the gastrointestinal tract by antibiotics. 80% of the immune system is housed in the gastrointestinal system and stabilized, in part, by the microbiome. I'll discuss the gastrointestinal system in chapter 9.

What is known as heat in TCM can be likened to overacidity in allopathic medicine. Overacidity breeds disease. Our cells thrive in an alkaline or balanced environment, and when there is too much acidity in our cells, they don't function properly.

Pathogens in the body also trigger the immune system to constantly defend itself, even if it can't. Examples of pathogens are viruses, parasites, fungi, and bacteria that don't belong in the body. Defending against them is part of our survival mechanism. As the immune system works endlessly, it generates inflammation, which is recognized in TCM as what is called "damp." In TCM, damp can be hot, cold, mixed, or other things, such as "wind."

In TCM, there is a mechanism to diagnose and treat these patterns naturally and effectively while strengthening the immune system. Knowing this mechanism helps us understand how diseases develop and how we can effectively address them and prevent them.

Acupuncture and Chinese Herbs Are Not Just for Backaches

Once patterns of disharmony are determined in a TCM evaluation, treatment can begin to restore the balance between *yin* and *yang* energies of the body to remedy a condition. This helps correct the root cause to treat it rather than just block the expression of the symptom.

In acupuncture, there are channels called meridians and collaterals that carry energy. This energy is moved through the body to maintain balance and feed the organs. This maintains body function. Along these channels are acupuncture points.

Acupuncture points can be verified with impedance meters to prove that they are, in fact, real. An impedance meter is an instrument that an electrician uses to detect electricity. Acupuncture points form groups with similar functions. We can combine certain acupuncture points to treat symptoms and patterns of disharmony causing those symptoms. This helps to treat the condition by restoring balance between the yin and yang energies of the body. Restoring balance eliminates symptoms naturally. Restoring balance also allows the body to recover from chronic illness over time and prevent other conditions from taking hold.

Acupuncture channels and points cannot be seen with the naked eye like blood vessels and nerves can. They are energetic points where energy enters or exits the body. They can be detected with point finders (impedance meters), which measure differences in energy across the skin. When a point finder goes over an acupuncture point, it "lights up" and measures the energy so we know that although we cannot see the acupuncture points and channels, they are definitely real. Remember that physicists are confirming that what appears to be a physical thing is just really dense energy. According to Albert Einstein, matter doesn't actually exist. Only energy exists.

It's well known that the human body emits several different forms of energy and this is the basis of the electrocardiogram (ECG) that cardiologists use to detect the electrical rhythm of the heart; thermography, which detects infra-red energy emitted by the body; and the EEG (electroencephalogram), used by neurologists to detect the electrical emissions of the brain. The electromagnetic field of the body can be measured by instruments called SQUIDs (Super conducting quantum interference devices).

When we understand Chinese medicine theory, we can strategically manipulate acupuncture points and restore balance by rebalancing the electromagnetic fields that regulate body function, helping a patient to feel much better.

The same can be accomplished with Chinese herbal formulas. Herbal formulas are groups of herbs put together specifically for their properties *when used together*. This combination of herbs is matched to specific patterns of disharmony that cause certain symptoms. Formulas can be customized for specific patterns of disharmony, so the best results can be achieved for an individual.

Chinese Herbs: Are they safe?

It's important to discuss the safety of Chinese herbs. With the dawn of the industrial revolution over a century ago, toxic metals began to seep into our soil, water and air and sadly, they've become ubiquitous finding their way into our food, drinking water, soil, prescription drugs and even Chinese herbal medicinals if precautions are not taken. Arsenic has been found in apples, rice and chicken. Lead and mercury have also found their way into our foods and medications. In response to this, many international governments have regulated the final products released to the public in all supplements, prescription drugs and herbal products. The international Good Manufacturing Practice (GMP) is a regulatory system for ensuring that products are consistently produced and controlled according to quality standards. GMP covers all aspects of production from the raw materials, production facilities, and equipment to the training and personal hygiene of staff. Detailed written procedures are necessary for each process that could affect the quality of the finished product. There must be systems to provide documented proof that correct procedures are consistently followed at each step in the manufacturing process every time a product is produced. It's important to make sure that any Chinese medicine practitioner who prescribes herbs for you is using Chinese herbs that are produced using GMP standards.

The theory behind Chinese herbal formulas is that each herb has qualities that are unique to it. Some herbs raise and lift energy, for example, while others cause drying. Other herbs are cooling or warming; some scatter energy. Different herbs enter different regions in the body. Some herbs can enter the heart, while others act on the liver. Some treat pain on the exterior of the body, and some open pores. The options go on and on. Knowing their unique qualities, you can combine herbs into a formula that suits the patterns of disharmony with precision, allowing for restoration of balance with minimal to no side effects.

The ancient Chinese physicians who devised Chinese herbal formulas determined their qualities by observing a plant or item in its natural environment. Flowers in general open outward and have a rising quality so in formulas that is, in fact, what they do.

Herbs such as shells have a sinking quality and help settle the mind by grounding it. An example of a shell used in TCM is Mu Li (oyster shell). It has salty and cool properties and is associated with the liver and kidney meridians. Its main functions are to calm the liver and suppress overactive *yang*, tranquilize the mind, arrest discharges, induce astringency, and soften hardness and nodules. It has sedative effects to settle the mind and ground it. It can help normalize blood pressure and treat insomnia for these reasons.

Some herbs, such as roots, are tonifying or strengthening. Roots are very grounding and give strength to a tree, so they do the same when ingested in the body. The Chinese herb Ci Wu Jia or Eleuthero (Siberian Ginseng) is a great example of a root herb. Used for thousands of years, Ci Wu Jia is used to invigorate qi (vital energy), strengthen and nourish the spleen and kidney energy systems. It's used in China to support general health and used for sleeplessness due to vivid dreams. It's pungent and slightly bitter in taste, energetically warming, and enters the spleen, kidney, and heart meridians. Generally, only the root is used. Ci Wu Jia is known as an adaptogen, which is a substance that strengthens the adrenal system, which is considered part of the kidney meridian in TCM. It's fascinating to think of the potential uses of Chinese herbal formulas!

Another great thing about Chinese herbal formulas is that the ancient Chinese physicians recognized that single herbs have some toxicity associated with them by the nature of what they do, so when making formulas, they took this into consideration and added other herbs to neutralize their toxicity. For example, the herb Cang Zhu (Black Atractylodis Rhizome) is used to treat dampness (inflammation) – it's drying by its nature and if used alone, it would eliminate inflammation by drying the patient out and cause problems related to dryness such as constipation or dry mouth. So, when making herbal formulas, they add balancing herbs to reduce this possibility. For example, a Chinese herbal formula called Ping Wei San (Calm the Stomach Powder) contains Cang Zhu as its principle herb but also contains Gan Cao (Rhizoma Glycyrrhizae) which harmonizes the formula preventing side effects. When a Chinese formula is matched to the correct pattern of disharmony, a balanced treatment without side effects and toxicity occurs. This is the reason why herbs are used in combination with other herbs and are rarely used as a single herb.

What does all this have to do with today's modern problems? In our modern world, the body is chronically stressed and undergoing unnecessary chemical reactions because it senses that there is a life-threatening event happening when there's not. The end result is that the body needlessly uses up a lot of *energy* — **qi and blood** — in the process.

This *energy* that TCM calls qi (pronounced chee) and blood that's being wasted during chronic stress can be in the form of hormones, vitamins, minerals, antioxidants, fats, proteins, and oxygen in needless chemical reactions that the body perceives are necessary for its survival as it continues to operate under the false notion that it's in fight-or-flight. The body usually cannot keep up with the demand for nutrients under these circumstances, and the body continues to activate survival mechanisms and goes after the next items on the food chain from which it can scavenge. These are its self-correcting forces at work. This helps the body assure that critical functions of heartbeat and breathing are maintained at the expense of other less important systems.

As the body hunts for what it needs by reducing blood flow to areas that are not critical - such as hair, skeletal muscles, bones, ovaries, and skin - we begin to experience hair loss, muscle loss, weight gain, osteoporosis, dry skin, rapid aging, menstrual irregularities, hot flashes, sleep disturbances, anxiety, fatigue, and even depression, just to name a few symptoms. And despite all this chaos, conventional medical testing is usually normal or non-specific at this point - the gray zone we previously discussed.

TCM however, reveals significant energy imbalances during this time, which can be found objectively with cellular and metabolic testing while blood work and conventional testing remains essentially normal.

When you begin to experience symptoms that linger, it's critical to remember these points and seek help from an integrative physician trained in traditional Chinese medicine to get to the root causes right away and fix them before trouble starts. In the next chapter, I'll explain the exciting new field of integrative medicine, which compliments TCM in a fascinating way.

CHAPTER EIGHT

INTEGRATIVE MEDICINE:

What is it?

Technically, integrative medicine is the integration, or mixing, of several different modalities to treat an individual as a whole. It endeavors to find the root cause of a condition to repair it rather than mask symptoms. It can combine conventional medicine with Chinese medicine or another system of medicine called functional medicine, which I'll explain later in this chapter.

Many integrative techniques combine mind-body methods such as yoga, meditation, massage, and biofeedback as part of their systems. In 2014, the American Board of Physicians and Surgeons formally recognized the field of integrative medicine as a formal medical specialty. I obtained my board certification in integrative medicine in 2017.

Treating Root Causes Versus Patching Up Symptoms

In my private practice, I use TCM as a hub to determine the root cause of symptoms. In TCM, many seemingly unrelated symptoms form patterns. For example, low back pain and night sweats are related in TCM, which indicates that the root cause of the problem is the energy system called kidney. This is to be contrasted from the organ that we call the kidney in conventional medicine because in Chinese medicine, systems are not anatomical entities but energy fields. In allopathic medicine, we don't relate night sweats and lower back pain, but in TCM they share a common pattern.

Night sweats can also be related to palpitations in TCM, which indicate that the root of the problem is in the energy field of the Heart. We wouldn't usually relate palpitations to night sweats in conventional medicine, but they go hand-in-hand in TCM.

Why is this important? In TCM, several symptoms can be tied together into patterns and treated at their root to resolve them faster rather than chasing around each individual symptom and targeting it separately. When we remember TCM theory, which says that the body is a fluid and integrated whole, this makes perfect sense.

The Gray Zone

I talked earlier about going to the doctor when you're not feeling well, only to be told there's nothing wrong. I call this the gray zone. The gray zone is that place where your bloodwork looks normal, but you feel horrible. Allopathic medicine usually has no answer for you at this point. If you go to the doctor long enough, you'll be prescribed an antidepressant, or worse, anxiety medication. I know because I used to do this based on my medical residency training.

When we look through the lens of integrative medicine by using functional medicine, however, there's a solution. We can determine a patient's status in the gray zone with a different type of test that can reveal what bloodwork cannot.

When the body goes into heavy compensation and begins to reshuffle resources, it steals from Paul to take to Peter so it will steal from the cells of the skeletal muscles, bones, ovaries, etc. to get what it needs. These specific cells are sacrificed so that cells more important for immediate survival (heart, lung and brain) get what they need to keep you alive. (See Figure 5).

The resources from certain cells in these lower priority areas form a type of buffer that protects the bloodstream to keep it normal and balanced. Meanwhile, these less important cells are deprived of critical nutrients they need for their functions and cause symptoms like fatigue, weight gain, chronic pain, and more. Keeping the bloodstream normal is critical to nourish the heart, lungs and brain. This is why blood work is usually normal in the "gray zone." What's the solution?

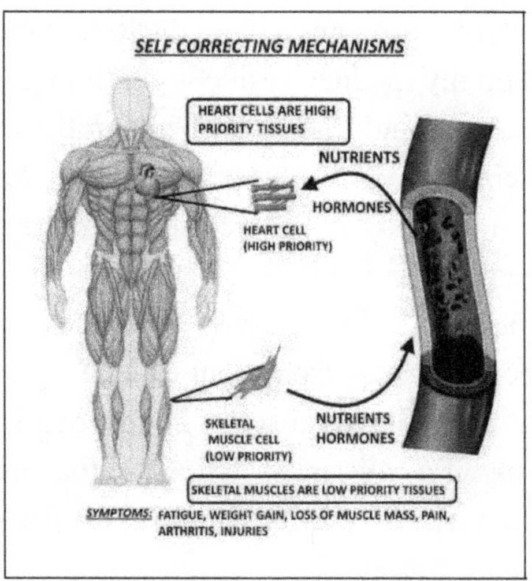

Figure 5: Under chronic stress, the body runs low on resources such as vitamins, minerals, proteins, and hormones. The body self-corrects to assure survival by taking these precious nutrients FROM low-priority tissues, such as skeletal muscle cells, and sends them TO high-priority tissues, such as heart cells. This mechanism assures survival by providing cells directly responsible for survival — such as heart, lung, and brainstem cells — with nutrients while depleting less important cells. This self-correcting mechanism leads to symptoms, such as loss of muscle mass, weight gain, fatigue, pain, arthritis, injuries, and hair loss.

Enter Functional Medicine

We can use this to our advantage in diagnosis by looking inside those so-called "less important" cells rather than in the bloodwork for answers. In functional medicine, this is a cornerstone of care. With modern analytics, cells can be cultivated in the lab and tested for darn near anything, including nutrient deficiencies and immune system responses, such as inflammation, hormone levels, metabolic disturbances, toxins, and more. The genes deep inside of cells can also be analyzed.

Total body storage of various nutrients, toxins, and hormones can also be approximated with urine testing. Testing the urine can also show us abnormalities in detoxification. For example, if I'd like to determine if a client is properly breaking down her estrogens, I can determine this with urinary analytes. This helps me support detoxification very specifically to reduce estrogen burden in the body.

Although testing is not part of TCM, in my private practice, I use TCM to target the type of testing I want to perform based on the patterns of disharmony, which describe the root causes of symptoms and conditions. I'm immediately aware of the root causes and can select the functional testing that will give me more information rather than using random testing to figure it out. For example, a patient may come in with fatigue and have damp accumulation and toxic heat based on my evaluation, which is a known cause of fatigue according to traditional Chinese medicine. I know at that point that I want to seek out toxins and sources of inflammation, and this guides my testing so it specifically targets the root cause of the condition.

I can anticipate that this patient likely has a heavy load of toxins or intolerances to certain things, such as foods or medications, for which I can test. This takes a lot of the guesswork out of the evaluation. Although TCM doesn't use testing, it's very powerful in the way that it helps target testing based in the patterns of disharmony. With TCM, we aren't stabbing in the dark and performing a bunch of tests to find out what's wrong. We already know what's wrong based on TCM and use the testing to target more comprehensive natural treatments.

For example, once those toxins are identified with the right testing, they can be successfully removed from the body. Repeat testing after an appropriate period of time can also confirm successful removal. TCM also helps us know if someone needs to be supported and strengthened before detoxification, which is very valuable because if we detox a patient who is depleted, he or she will only get weaker, and those toxins will build up again. (See Figure 6).

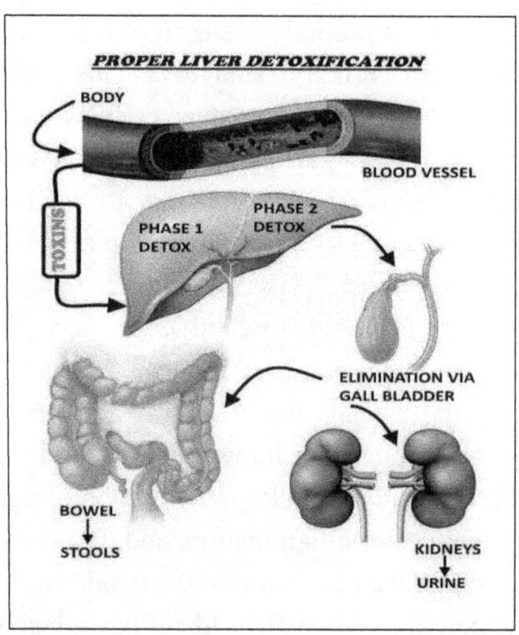

Figure 6: Detoxification occurs throughout the body; however, the liver is principally responsible for detoxification of all substances that enter the bloodstream such as food, chemicals, and medications. There are two phases of detoxification. Phase 1 transforms toxins into forms that can be further broken down in Phase 2. This occurs via a series of enzymes called cytochrome P450. Phase 2 involves conjugation, which attaches water-soluble substances to help shuttle toxins into bile and urine to be eliminated from the body.

The combination of TCM as a guiding principle and main treatment combined with cutting edge cellular-based testing is a powerful method of integrative medicine I utilize with my private clients to treat most conditions and symptoms. Integrative medicine can successfully help improve and prevent most chronic conditions such as heart disease, diabetes, Alzheimer's dementia, autism, cancer, and more.

It can help reduce the need for synthetic drugs and help the body heal from the impact of these toxins. Integrative techniques use more natural options that are proven safe and effective. The reason this is possible is because TCM and functional/integrative medicine specifically diagnose the underlying patterns and causes of conditions and treat from this perspective. The need to treat the underlying cause of symptoms and conditions can't be emphasized enough. It's the key to wellness.

Cindy, a 45-year-old mother of two, came to my office complaining of fatigue, weight gain, and low sex drive after seeing two other physicians. Her symptoms started three years prior to seeing me, and her bloodwork and preventive screening tests were always normal. Cindy exercised five days a week and restricted her calories during those three years and actually gained weight! She had standard bloodwork for the complaint of fatigue, weight gain, and low libido which consisted of blood cell counts, thyroid stimulating hormone, free T4, blood levels of testosterone, estrogen, progesterone, blood sugar, cholesterol, liver and kidney function testing.

All of these results were always normal, and her doctors told her to accept it as part of aging. Luckily, Cindy knew that something was wrong and kept searching for answers, and she came to see me. My TCM-based evaluation of Cindy indicated kidney and liver meridian deficiencies. Knowing the cause of Cindy's symptoms prompted me to ask Cindy to reduce her activities and eat foods that were more nourishing for her particular pattern of disharmony. I asked her to do restorative yoga or tai chi instead of the draining boot camp workouts she was doing. I asked her to cut out dairy and wheat and to eat cooked leafy and root vegetables, soups and bone broths. I increased her protein and fat intake as well.

Since the causes of her symptoms were related to the liver and kidney meridians, I tested Cindy's *cellular* levels of hormones and nutrients, which revealed the following:

- significant adrenal fatigue (low DHEA, low progesterone)
- suboptimal thyroid function with low free T3, normal T4, and TSH
- carnitine deficiency
- oleic acid deficiency
- B12 deficiency
- Pantothenic acid deficiency
- Zinc deficiency
- Glutathione deficiency

I added foods rich in the nutrients to which she was deficient to her nutrition plan. I prescribed bioidentical DHEA (an adrenal hormone), bioidentical progesterone, and adaptogenic herbs to support the adrenal glands. I optimized Cindy's thyroid with the nutrients in which she was deficient. Cindy was iodine-deficient based on urine testing so I prescribed low dose iodine to correct this. We eventually started her on combined natural thyroid replacement therapy as well.

At Cindy's one-month follow-up, she was happy to report that her energy was much better and she had lost seven pounds. Cindy was well on her way to feeling better because her body function was able to improve on a *cellular* and metabolic level. Her bloodwork didn't reveal any of the hormone or nutrient deficiencies that her cellular-based testing revealed. Had Cindy not taken these extra steps while in the gray zone, she would've kept gaining weight and remained tired until diagnosed with other more significant conditions or diseases later. Cindy is another valuable example of the power of energy-based medical integration to make a significant difference in someone's life quickly and have incredible value long-term, even when conventional medicine can't find anything wrong.

The reasons why traditional Chinese medicine (TCM) and functional medicine are invaluable to our wellness are better understood once we have a clear understanding of why bloodwork deceives us. I'll discuss this in the next chapter.

CHAPTER NINE

LIES YOUR BLOODWORK TOLD YOU

As the body becomes more and more stressed, it needs to maintain critical tasks, such as heartbeat and brain function. It does so in an ingenious way that leads us to believe that all is well when, in fact, all hell is about to break loose. Stress is the ultimate root cause of all symptoms and disease as we've discussed. Under stress, your body utilizes a lot more energy than it would without stress. This leads to a supply/demand mismatch leading to various nutrient and hormone deficits. Levels of vitamins, antioxidants, minerals, and proteins like hormones and enzymes all begin to decline as the body scrambles to keep up with the demands for energy utilization to perform its functions. As the supply of nutrients and hormones declines, the body begins to make choices that are based in the need for immediate survival. Remember its #1 job is to keep you alive by keeping your heart beating, your lungs breathing, and the brain synapses firing to control that breathing and heartbeat. This is part of the fight-or-flight mechanism that's hardwired in your body. As you run low on energy, you naturally feel more tired and less rested.

Your metabolism drops and you may gain weight. These are signs that your body is beginning to shuffle its resources to maintain critical body functions at the expense of less critical functions. Under these circumstances, maintenance of body weight and hair growth just isn't at the top of the survival list. Having extra energy to have sex, exercise, or think clearly doesn't make it to the top of the priority list either. As we begin to experience this fatigue, weight gain, hair loss, and low sex drive and bring this up to our primary care physicians, we're often left without answers, or worse, we're told this is a normal part of aging.

In allopathic medicine, bloodwork is a cornerstone of diagnosis of disease. Many of us have experienced not feeling well and have gone to the doctor only to be told that everything is normal. Why is that? As we now know, your body is a brilliant machine and knows that the bloodstream feeds the heart, lungs, and brain, which are critical for body function and survival. ***It's through the blood stream that all cells of the heart, lungs and brain receive oxygen and nutrients they need to live.***

The body knows it had better maintain normal blood function and flow to keep you alive. If your blood levels of potassium, or sodium are abnormal, you can have heart failure. If your blood can't carry oxygen to critical systems like your heart or brain, you can die of a heart attack or stroke. Guess what'll happen if you look in the bloodstream for a problem when you're tired, gaining weight and losing hair? The body goes to great lengths to "normalize" the blood stream to keep you alive. You won't find significant abnormalities in the blood work until you've had symptoms so long you finally do have a disease.

If your bloodstream can't carry necessary nutrients and oxygen to other less critical but important systems, poor body function initially manifested as fatigue, weight gain, low sex drive, can progress to diseases that can eventually become life-threatening, such as diabetes or heart disease.

When the body can no longer maintain normal blood function and flow, critical bodily functions cannot be maintained. The body still prioritizes under these circumstances to make sure the heart, brain and lungs get what they need, but your *immune system, gastrointestinal system, ovaries/testes, hair follicles, joints, and bones will likely not get their fair share*. And once the body begins to decompensate in this way, it can be like a domino effect. Once one system stops working properly, several others follow suit because as it's known in TCM, the body is an integrated dynamic whole.

It may only take a cold to start a cascade of symptoms that cause someone to spiral out during menopause. I hear this all the time from my new patients. They were doing just fine until a stressful event happened. They caught a cold or lost a job; suddenly they got one symptom after another and felt terrible. They may even be diagnosed with multiple conditions in a row. Once the body loses its ability to compensate, it spirals down quickly if there's no intervention to fix the root causes and re-stabilize it.

Many get trapped in the allopathic medicine cycle and get prescribed antidepressants, antibiotics, anxiety medications, and sleeping pills unnecessarily in an attempt to help these symptoms. Since these treatments don't address the root cause, which is the impact of stress on the body, the cycle of disease and symptoms rolls on unabated for many.

Blocking symptom expression in the body is equivalent to putting your finger in the hole in a dam. While the water stops leaking for the moment, you didn't really fix the problem so another leak will soon follow. Symptoms are part of the body's defense mechanism to let you know it's struggling or out of balance in some way. When the body's defense mechanism is disturbed through symptom blocking, the problem still exists so it must compensate and express in a different way. This is another reason medications have side effects. The symptom was masked, the root cause was not addressed, and the problem is still present in the body. The medications further destabilize of the body resulting in side effects.

The body will never shut down its fight-or-flight response because it's embedded in its function for survival. Instead, the body will seek to sound the alarm in a different way until it's heard loud and clear. *If the root cause of symptoms is not successfully addressed the sounding of the alarm may come in the form of a heart attack or diagnosis of cancer.*

When bloodwork doesn't explain the cause of symptoms it's critical to use TCM to reverse the downward spiral. During this time, it's critical to be on the right nutrition and lifestyle plans that address these root causes in a personalized fashion. Chinese herbal formulas, targeted nutrition, and acupuncture work very well at this stage long before diseases have set in.

The use of bloodwork for evaluation of symptoms misses certain conditions and energy imbalances present in the body. These energy imbalances take place inside the body's cells, where critical body functions take place. The concurrent use of cellular-based testing with TCM to determine the root causes provides powerful ammunition to correct these underlying causes so the body can stop sounding the alarm and have balance and harmony.

Body Economics: The Basics of Supply and Demand

The body has a limited supply of resources that must be replenished daily for proper body function. Remember the second law of thermodynamics clearly tells us that systems break down over time if left unattended. Energy must be pumped back in to maintain the system and prevent breakdown. The blood stream is a means by which to carry these nutrients and energy to the cells of the body. We can liken the blood stream to a transportation highway. Not much is really functioning in the blood stream until it reaches and enters the body's cells. When demand outweighs supply, certain cells of the body sacrifice their resources to the blood stream so these critical nutrients can get to more important cells. *So, the blood stream, by default, tends to have more nutrients and oxygen flowing through it to get to important cells and this leads to the false perception that all is well even in the presence of significant symptoms.*

There are many reasons why demand outweighs supply in the body, leading to deficiency of significant amounts of nutrients. Our food supply is increasingly devoid of minerals and vitamins; multiple studies have confirmed this. Our gastrointestinal tracts have been assaulted by pesticides and processed foods. A survey conducted by New York University found that an astounding 74% of Americans have gastrointestinal symptoms such as bloating, gas, diarrhea, or constipation. Studies also confirm that 20% of the U.S. population has a *significant* gastrointestinal **disease** like ulcerative colitis or Crohn's disease, which can open the door to other significant diseases like cancer.

Lack of sleep is another reason why demand outweighs supply. When we don't sleep sufficiently, our bodies are "on" more than they should be. This creates increased demand. When the body is taken out of rhythm, it compensates to a point, but we have forced the body to compensate to the point where it runs out of gas, causing chronic diseases, and even death. Always remember the second law of thermodynamics - *you have to put back in what you take out*.

In the next chapter, I'll discuss how this all comes together in my unifying theory of disease – what I believe underlies all diseases.

CHAPTER TEN

A UNIFYING THEORY OF DISEASE FORMATION AND PREVENTION

The idea that diseases are random or unrelated to each other is deeply flawed. There are critical common threads that should be explored in order to provide a path out of the disaster that is our current sickness care paradigm. The first step is to understand the basics of body function. We take body function for granted because the body performs them seamlessly. Our hearts beat, lungs breathe, eyes see and our ears hear without effort. There's a lot more body function than what we recognize. The reason our body can produce these functions is due to its cells and how they communicate with each other. We have between 70 trillion to 100 trillion cells in our bodies. There are billions of chemical reactions going on in each cell at any given moment – day and night.

Cellular functions range from heartbeat, breathing, movement, reproduction, digestion, energy production, vision, hearing, feeling, moving, smelling, temperature regulation, hair growth, tasting, DNA/gene repair and reproduction, immunity, and thinking. These functions are fueled by energy production *inside* the cells. Cells then use this energy currency to power the chemical reactions that result in body functions. For example, your eye cells have to make their own energy from the inside and then use this energy to power the chemical reactions that allow you to see color, shades of gray, and night vision. Even eye lubrication is powered by this energy made inside of cells. Cells make their energy using what are called mitochondria via a series of chemical reactions known as the Krebs or Citric Acid Cycle. The Krebs Cycle uses the fats, proteins, and carbohydrates (polysaccharides) from the foods we eat and converts them into the energy currency of the body called ATP (adenosine triphosphate) through the use of oxygen. All the cells in the body use ATP to power **all** body functions. Nothing happens in the body without ATP being used as the energy currency to produce it. I'll discuss the mechanisms cells use to make this precious energy later in this chapter.

SELF CORRECTING FORCES, FOOD CHAINS AND GRAY ZONES

Everything in nature is part of a food chain. A food chain is how energy flows from one living organism or system to another. What we see in nature is also reflected within our bodies. This is very prevalent in Eastern philosophies: "As above, so below." In other words, what we see around us is also happening inside of us. Inside the body, a food chain is how energy flows from one system or group of cells to another. The body regulates energy flow very tightly and assures that the most important cells get energy before less important cells.

Even the different parts of the brain are on a food chain! The inner most cells of the brain called the brain stem have extremely high priority because they're directly responsible for controlling heartbeat and breathing! This is why they get first dibs on the blood flow into the brain from the heart. The brain cells that are more closer to the periphery of the brain or cerebral hemispheres are not as important for immediate survival. This is where memory is stored and behavior and mood are regulated, for example. If there aren't enough nutrients and resources for the entire brain, the body will decide which brain cells get these precious resources and leave the cells on the periphery of the brain more vulnerable. This leads to poor concentration, memory loss, mood disorders and can even be a cause of Alzheimer dementia as illustrated in figure 7.

So why do some people get Alzheimer's dementia and others don't? What determines the specific disease you may get varies for everyone and this is where genetic predisposition or possibly traumatic injury to certain areas of the body may play a role. If you injure an area that's responsible for certain functions, there may be poor nutrient and oxygen circulation in that area leading to an increased risk of disease there. This is a well understood mechanism for arthritis.

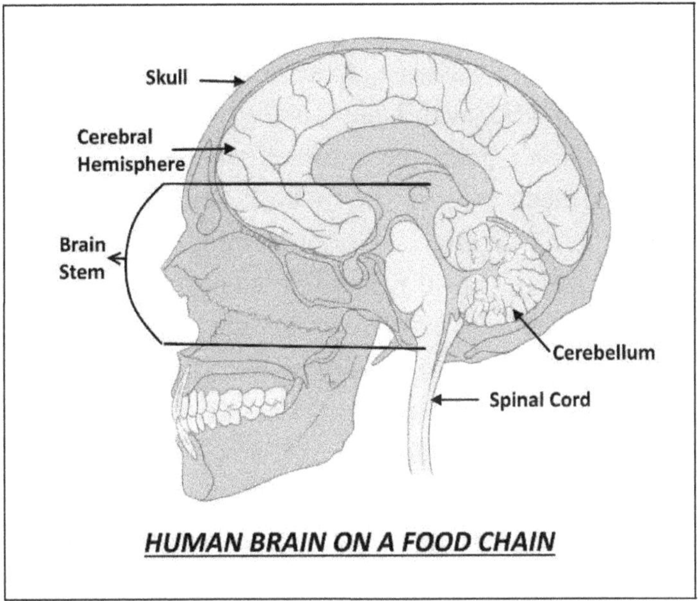

Figure 7: This illustration shows a cross-section of the human head, which houses the brain. Deep in the center of the brain is the brainstem, which controls critical body functions necessary for life such as breathing and heartbeat. The main blood vessels that come into the brain deliver nutrients and oxygen to the brainstem as a top priority for survival. The cerebral hemispheres are located in the outer regions of the brain and control movement, memory, speech, emotions, reading, writing, and learning. These functions are not critical for immediate survival, and the regions of the brain that control them are more on the periphery of the brain. When there are not enough nutrients to go around, the periphery gets less supply so the brainstem can get sufficient nutrition and oxygen. This survival mechanism may result in brain tumors, Alzheimer's dementia, or even Autism in children.

Injury to a joint can easily lead to poor oxygenation or nutrient distribution in that joint which results in inflammation and degeneration of cartilage and other connective tissues in the immediate area. However, if after the injury, steps are taken to restore proper nutrient and oxygen delivery to that area, we can drastically reduce the incidence of arthritis. I was a high school and collegiate basketball player and tore the medial meniscus in my right knee after my first year of college basketball. I had an MRI and I was told by the orthopedic surgeon that I should expect to have arthritis in my right knee by the time I reached 30 years of age. I told myself that day that there was NO WAY I was going to get arthritis and decided that I was going to heal my knee with heat, a brace to avoid further injury and strength training to build the muscles around my knee for better support. I continued to work on my knee with acupuncture, infrared heat therapy, and Chinese herbs after learning about these modalities later in my career just as a preventive measure. To this day, I have absolutely no pain or inflammation, and no restrictions in my activities. If I'd listened to the orthopedic surgeon, I would've had surgery on my knee and probably would have arthritis by now. Thankfully I was guided in another direction!

If you have a genetic predisposition to Alzheimer's dementia, you may be more likely to be afflicted if you have more lactic acid buildup and damage to brain cells as a result of not getting enough nutrients and oxygen into those brain cells for proper function. Although many other parts of your body may be deprived of oxygen and nutrients, the genetic predisposition to Alzheimer's dementia will make it easier for these symptoms to manifest as short-term memory loss consistent with Alzheimer's dementia. You can use this awareness for prevention. It stands to reason based on simple physiological principles, that if we assure that the Kreb's Cycle is working properly, we can avoid Alzheimer's dementia, even in the face of genetic predisposition. This is well known in the field of epigenetics. Epigenetics is about what's going on around your genes as they sit inside your cells. It's all about the cellular environment and how genes respond to those signals they get from the inside of your cells. If nutrients and oxygen are missing, your genes will respond very differently than if the inside of your cells are nutritionally sound. Why?

Our body's self-correcting mechanism knows that our hair follicles are not as important as our heart cells. We can survive being bald, but we can't survive without a heartbeat. It knows that our bones are not as important as our brain which is why we can survive with osteoporosis, but we can't survive without blood flow to our brain. Our body very slowly shunts blood away from low-priority cells to send it to high-priority cells under chronic stress. In other words, our body reshuffles its resources to keep the peace. We see extreme examples of this real-life situation while watching medical dramas on TV: the car crash and the victim with internal bleeding, for example. The medical staff whisks him into the ER; he looks extremely pale, his lips are blue, and he may be unconscious because he's losing blood fast. His skin is pale and his lips are blue because the body has instantaneously shunted blood flow to the internal critical organs such as the heart and brain, and away from the non-critical areas such as skin, bones, and muscles. This is a survival mechanism to maintain blood flow to the heart and brain which is very well recognized in medicine.

Chronic stress is no different from the above example, except that *its effects occur so slowly over an extended period of time that we don't immediately notice them.* We see this with undiagnosed colon cancer in certain patients, for example. Many people with undiagnosed colon cancer have internal bleeding, but it's so slow that it's not noticeable until it's been happening for a long time and comes up during a random blood test that shows that the patient is severely anemic, but he may not even be aware of it. This is another example of blood work being normal until it's too late. The body's had time to compensate and keep the peace so the person with colon cancer won't feel dizzy or pass out like the car crash victim.

In the example of the car crash victim who's bleeding fast, the body doesn't have time to compensate so it has to adapt quickly. That person will have dizziness, weakness, and may even pass out due to rapid blood loss. The patient who had the car accident may have bloodwork that reveals the same blood count as the person with colon cancer, who has minimal or no symptoms. In both of these extreme examples, the situation was so dire that the blood work became abnormal as an indication that a severe condition exists. In the case of the colon cancer patient, he may have no symptoms despite abnormal blood work. The colon cancer patient's blood work would be normal despite the presence of cancer until he becomes anemic from the blood loss.

In other cases, the blood work may remain normal even in the presence of significant symptoms. For example, in the case of Jane in chapter 2, she had a severe small bowel infection and multiple cellular nutrient deficiencies, but her blood work was completely normal. Why does the body do this? Why is the blood stream such an inconsistent indicator of our health? The body's main concern is to keep us alive. To do this, it must provide blood flow with critically needed oxygen and nutrients to the heart, brain and lungs. When we look in the blood stream, we'll capture a falsely normal environment that reflects what the body is prioritizing to the heart, brain and lungs. The findings in the *blood work* will be completely different than what we find in the *cells* of lower priority areas such as hair follicles, bones, and immune cells who are being deprived of what they need. The ability of the body to do this is absolutely essential because otherwise, we'd die from stress.

The fight-or-flight mechanism was designed for life-threatening situations, such as being attacked by predators when we appeared on Earth 200,000 years ago. It's designed to instantly raise blood pressure and heart rate to get the body prepared to run or fight for survival.

Another fight-or-flight function is to make sure that our body doesn't stop to eliminate waste through urination or bowel movements by shunting blood flow away from the kidneys and bowels, so we can fight or flee from harm if being chased by a bear. We wouldn't get very far if we had to stop to urinate while a hungry bear was chasing us. It also allows for the critical organs responsible for our immediate safety to get all the oxygen and nutrients they need to support the fight-or-flight mechanism.

This survival mechanism also knows to shut down reproduction during times of threat from predators so that our young are not eaten alive. It protects our reproductive energy in ingenious ways! Back then, the circumstances under which the fight or flight mechanism kicked in either resulted in immediate death or survival. There wasn't much in between. We either ran away from the predator or were eaten alive. Either way, the fight-or-flight mechanism wasn't active for long. We've come a long way and no longer have major predators. We're closer to the top of the food chain so the body shouldn't be in survival mode, should it? No, it shouldn't, but it's been *forced to continue to believe it's being threatened by the unprecedented chronic stress that we experience in our modern lifestyle*.

Our body functions from within its cells, which are its basic building blocks. There are up to 100 trillion cells in the human body undergoing trillions of chemical reactions day and night to maintain body function. These cells don't have brains or eyes, and they can't tell one kind of stress from another kind of stress. In other words, they don't know if we're angry because we're stuck in traffic or if we're panicking because we're being chased by a bear. We *as individuals*, of course, know because we have a brain, and we can talk ourselves down after assessing the situation to determine if it's life-threatening or not, but our 100 trillion cells don't have a clue. They *receive the same chemical signals of stress whether it's a life-threatening situation or not* because this is a system that originated over 200,000 years ago, and it hasn't changed at all.

As our cells are constantly overworking and reacting to stress, they run out of precious resources. Modern-day stress is like driving your car around but never turning off the engine. Imagine leaving your car in the garage with the engine running all the time; you would blow your engine. Your body's cells are no different with one critically important difference: our bodies are much more sophisticated than our cars! As important cells start to run low on resources - such as proteins, fats, vitamins, minerals, hormones, and enzymes - the body's self-correcting mechanisms kick in and shuffle resources around. Even the most sophisticated cars can't do that! The body takes resources from low-priority cells to high-priority cells. While this is life-saving, it also leaves those low-priority cells drained and worn out.

Cells have a warning system as they run out of resources and lose function: we call this warning system our symptoms! Some symptoms may include fatigue, weight gain, anxiety, depression, achy joints and muscles, abnormal menstruation, inflammation, and memory loss to name a few. Even our immune and gastrointestinal systems, as important as they are, *aren't as important* as the heart and brain for *immediate* survival. Our skeletal muscle cells like our calves and biceps are not very important if high-priority cells like our heart and brain cells need resources. In fact, our skeletal muscle cells are a great source of energy and protein to keep our body going in an emergency. Our body begins to break down our muscle cells to retrieve some of that energy and protein. The problem is that our muscle cells help us burn energy as part of our metabolism, too, so when our body loses muscle mass under stress, we may develop symptoms such as weight gain and tiredness.

With the onset of symptoms of fatigue, weight gain, poor concentration, and aches and pains, we're in a **gray zone**. Our bloodwork and other diagnostic testing would come back normal if we went to our doctor's office to complain about these symptoms. *Allopathic medicine doesn't have testing in place to reveal what our body needs at this critical stage because its goal is to diagnose disease* and, in the gray zone, you don't yet have a disease, so not much is found in our allopathic model.

The gray zone is critical because if the body can get what it needs at this point, these symptoms go away, and more importantly, we unknowingly prevent diseases that eventually come from the cellular dysfunction that caused these symptoms in the first place. One important lesson I've learned is that the body doesn't waste its energy. In other words, it doesn't produce symptoms for the sake of producing symptoms. *Symptoms are the body's means of communicating in an effort to correct itself because it can't do so on its own.*

Gray Zone, Land of Possibilities: Wellness or Disease?

When the body perceives stress, it continues to undergo fight of flight responses as we discussed above. The gray zone is the zone where we know something is wrong, but conventional allopathic medicine can't identify what it is, or it finds some things and treats them, but our symptoms persist.

This is a critical time for intervention, but what can we do when we keep going to the doctor, and we're told nothing is wrong? We're at a tipping point. Either we can correct the abnormalities before they become diseases, or we can keep waiting until our bloodwork and conventional diagnostic studies head south, and we actually do have a disease. Although diseases seem to come out of nowhere, my clients are often surprised to find out that normal body function, symptoms, and diseases are on the same spectrum. There's a considerable amount of time between having normal body function and being diagnosed with a disease and there's a lot going on under the radar that we can't see with allopathic evaluation and testing. Knowing you're in the gray zone provides a great opportunity for intervention to reverse the course *if you know what to do*. The following figure illustrates this spectrum from normal to disease. (See figure 8).

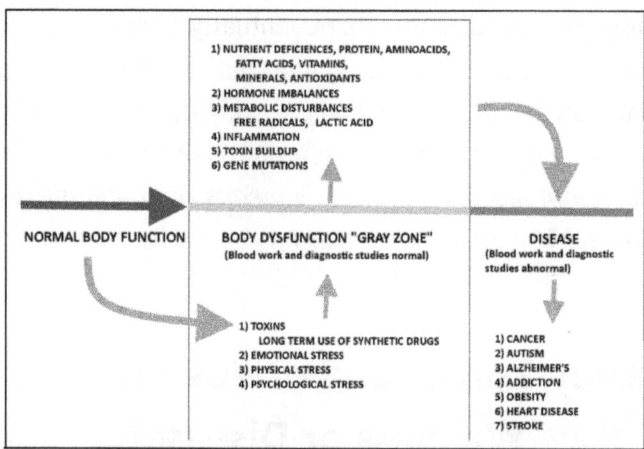

Figure 8: The body isn't normal one day and diseased the next. This illustration shows the progression from normal body function to disease onset and the steps that go undetected along the way in the "gray zone." As the body is chronically exposed to synthetic drugs, toxins, and other stressors— whether emotional, physical, or psychological — the body moves along the spectrum towards disease. In the gray zone, blood work and diagnostic testing is normal despite symptoms. TCM can diagnose energy imbalances in the body during this time that conventional medicine cannot. Hidden inside the cells, we can detect nutrient deficiencies, hormone imbalances, metabolic disturbances, and inflammation as depicted here. As the body endures these cellular disturbances over time, it keeps moving along the spectrum towards diseases which are finally detectable by conventional means such as blood work and diagnostic studies years later.

TCM allows for diagnosis and treatment in the gray zone. Traditional Chinese medicine looks at the energy of the body and finds patterns of imbalance in that energy, which we can correct to restore the body's relationship with itself and its environment to achieve harmony. The human body is made of energy converted to mass: $E = mc^2$. There's energy that we can't see with our "senses" that is diagnosable with TCM. In fact, physicists now tell us with certainty that only 1% of the universe is made of matter. Even what we think is physical is mostly space consisting of unfathomable energy. The tiny little atoms that make up what we think are physical structures are 99% space and energy. Our bodies are no different, mostly made of space and energy.

Although not an energy-based system of medicine, functional medicine also allows for some diagnosis and treatment in that gray zone. While functional medicine is technically anatomical and deductive, it looks in the cells for answers and reveals significant dysfunction when bloodwork remains normal. My clients are often shocked by what we find in their cells after recently having normal blood work. The cellular-based testing done in the field of functional medicine doesn't answer all that's needed, but it's a great addition to help complement what TCM reveals. *Together these two modalities are extremely powerful to treat root causes of symptoms and reverse the risk of disease.*

Energy: The Secret Sauce of Body Function

The cornerstone of wellness is the body's ability to make, use and distribute energy with flawless precision. The body is remarkably well equipped to perform these functions *if* it has the tools to make it happen. As we've discussed, the average person has 70 trillion to 100 trillion cells working flawlessly together. Within each cell, there are trillions of chemical reactions going on. This is what allows us to move, see, smell, think, reproduce, digest, eliminate waste, fight infections, hear, read this book, and much more. Mitochondria are referred to as "power houses" because these are where the vast majority of energy called ATP (adenosine triphosphate) is made in all cells. Most cells each contain 1000-2000 mitochondria. (See figure 9.)

The mitochondria inside our cells are critical and we wouldn't exist without these structures inside all our cells. The more energy the cells use, the more mitochondria they have. For example, the heart which is at the top of the food chain in the body, has the most mitochondria of any organ in the body! The heart beats up to 115,000 times a day, day after day, year after year and decade after decade, with no breaks!

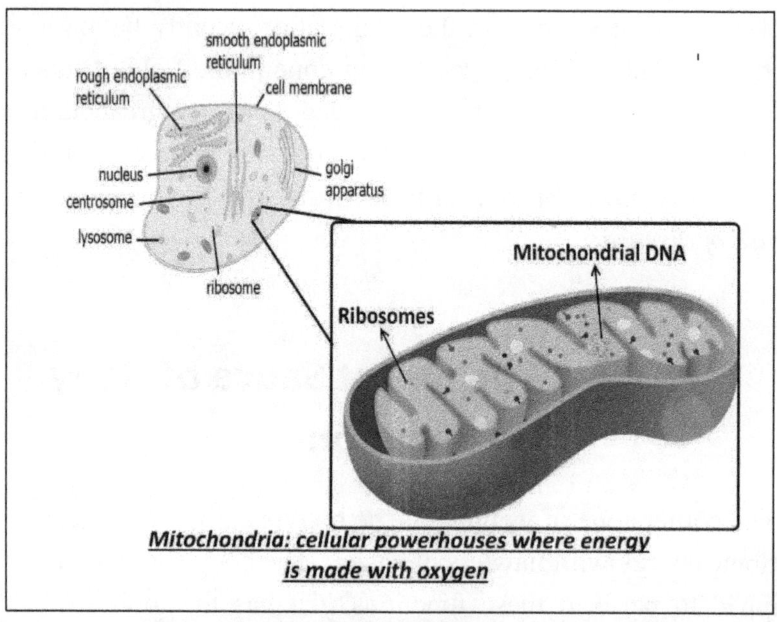

Figure 9: Mitochondria are located inside the body's cells. Mitochondria are where cellular energy is made. The currency of the body's cells is called ATP (adenosine triphosphate). Cells that require a lot of energy such as heart muscles and skeletal muscles contain much more mitochondria than cells that use less energy, such as hair follicles and skin cells. Mitochondria are very delicate and can be easily damaged.

That demands a ton of energy and the mitochondria are there cranking out energy in the form of ATP at all times. Although you may think such a critical function would take up all the mitochondria's time, they have two other critical functions:

1. programmed cell death called apoptosis
2. reproduction and division of mitochondria

Programmed cell death called apoptosis is an important function of our cells. Normally, cells are "born," they perform their functions, they reproduce and divide to create other fresh cells to take over these functions, then they are *programmed* to die. The immune system then calls the clean-up crew to remove the dead cell from the body to be replaced by a shiny new cell. This assures that our body function can remain normal and we don't have worn out cells underperforming. This is also a critical mechanism to prevent cancer. Cancer, by definition, is the loss of programmed cell death. Cancer is an immortal cell, a cell that has lost its programming to die, which then slowly reproduces and divides leading to other immortal cells. This dire malfunction stays under the radar for years as it accumulates more and more cells. After a few years, there are billions of immortal cells that finally become a visible mass on examination or a radiological study like an X-ray, CT scan, or MRI. Mitochondria are critical control points for the prevention of cancer and the assurance of proper body function.

Mitochondria also contain specific genes in their DNA to reproduce themselves. In other words, mitochondria are responsible for their own reproduction independent of the genes that are responsible for cellular reproduction. The cell's nucleus houses these other genes that are responsible for the cell's reproduction. Communication between the mitochondria and nucleus of each cell is critical for control of that cell's programmed death and reproduction.

This communication is maintained by the production of a molecule called NAD or nicotinamide adenine dinucleotide, and is critical for the exchange of electrons involved in the making of ATP, the body's energy currency. When this happens **inside** the mitochondria where it's meant to happen, it's called **aerobic** respiration or the making of energy *with* oxygen, which results in much more energy than if it's made **outside** the mitochondria. NAD is being proven in numerous studies to have significant anti-aging properties for this very reason! You'll look, feel, and literally BE much younger if your mitochondria can crank out energy and help your cells renew themselves. This is anti-aging by definition! Aging occurs when cells can't make ample energy to support their functions resulting in damage to the cells and mitochondria! True to form, the body actually has a back-up ready in case it can't make adequate energy as we'll discuss next.

When the body is unable to make energy with oxygen due to metabolic damage or oxidative stress, energy is made OUTSIDE of the mitochondria resulting in a *dangerous* buildup of lactic acid and alcohol, and much less NAD and ATP is made. This is called **anaerobic** respiration and is a backup in case the mitochondria are damaged, or the body is in some type of metabolic distress. (See Figure 10.)

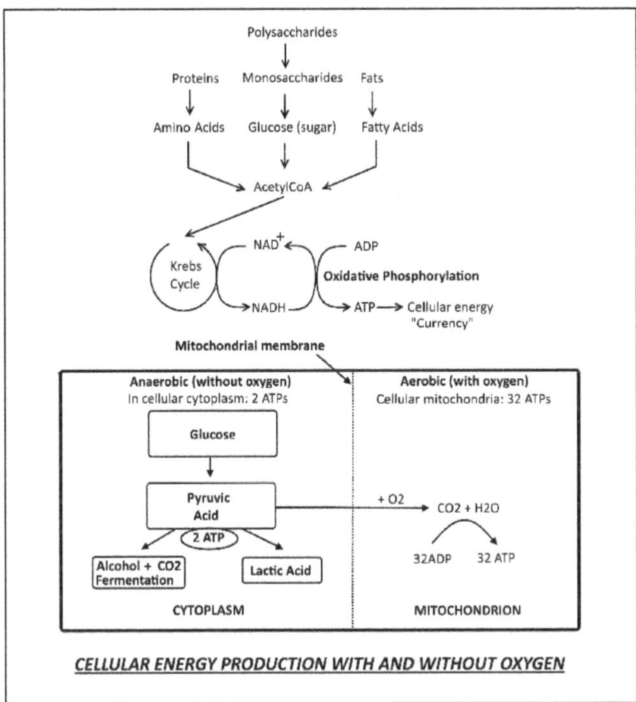

Figure 10: KREBS (CITRIC ACID) CYCLE: This illustration demonstrates how the mitochondria use our food and break it down into its basic components to make energy via a complex series of chemical reactions called the Krebs Cycle. Whether or not a cell has oxygen available makes a huge difference in the amount of energy the mitochondria can produce. Without oxygen, mitochondria can only make two (2) units of ATP per molecule of glucose; whereas with oxygen they can make 32 units of ATP with that same molecule of glucose. This has a direct impact on our metabolism and our ability to make and use energy. Stress in the form of toxins and nutrient deficiencies can disrupt this critical function of our mitochondria.

You will NOT look, feel, and BE younger when this happens. The problem with this back-up system is that it's not meant to be on all the time. That's why it's a backup and not the main attraction. It's for emergencies only because the body can't function normally that way for long, but it gives the body time to correct the malfunction. It's akin to the adage "In Case of Emergency Break Glass" to pull the fire alarm. It's not something we should have to do daily, but in our 21st century pressure cooker, that's exactly what we're doing on a cellular level and this is why the body can't repair itself and spirals downhill straight towards rapid aging and dangerous diseases. If the body can't repair itself, it adapts the best it can by initiating a cascade of reactions to compensate for the lack of energy and inability to perform vital functions.

For example, cells that can't get enough oxygen and make enough energy turn on a gene to adapt to this lack of oxygen called HIF or hypoxia-inducing factor which helps the body to make energy, but a lot less than normal. This gene activation leads to the activation of a cascade of other genes that **lead to cancer cell formation**. Why does the body set up such a dire backup system? Ultimately, if the body has to choose between having a broad lack of oxygen and energy production in crucial cells like the heart and brain versus allowing the formation of cancer cells in order to make some energy rather than none, it will pick cancer cell formation every time. Why? Your body's self-correcting forces know that cancer doesn't kill you immediately, but a heart attack or stroke is much more immediately deadly. Additionally, cells that can't get enough oxygen also produce more blood vessels in an attempt to get more oxygen. This increase of blood vessels also happens to fuel cancer cells. So, the body ends up in a vicious circle due to its inability to get what it needs to function. This mechanism isn't just responsible for cancer cell formation. It may also be responsible for Autism, Alzheimer's, autoimmune diseases, and even drug addiction! It's important to remember that the body's self-correcting forces will accept any of the above diseases over a heart attack or stroke if it has to choose. Why? Because the above diseases are not immediately life-threatening whereas a heart attack or stroke is immediately life-threatening. This doesn't mean that the body is immune to heart attacks and strokes. They're at the top of the list as causes of death. As the body continues to struggle, eventually these more crucial functions are also impeded leading to these deadly strokes and heart attacks. It's very likely that these people are metabolic disasters with significant cellular abnormalities long before they have a heart attack or stroke, but allopathic medicine doesn't look for these anomalies so it appears that the heart attack occurred out of the blue when it was years in the making as the body's self-correcting systems struggled under the radar to keep the peace.

Although the exact details of these compensation or self-correcting mechanisms aren't clear, what is clear is that the normal function of the cells CAN and MUST be restored to protect against diseases such as cancer, heart attacks, strokes, and Alzheimer's dementia. If we can restore proper cellular energy production and function, we can successfully treat symptoms that can lead to diseases, thereby preventing them altogether.

Harvard University recently published what they are coining as an "anti-aging" discovery in the March 2017 edition of *Science* magazine. They showed that *DNA could be repaired* in rats by exposing rats to the building blocks of NAD, a component of the Krebs cycle that mitochondria use to make ATP energy. In other words, when the rats' mitochondria were able to complete the Krebs cycle and make energy, damaged genes were repaired! This is critical because the Krebs cycle is involved in just about every single body function conceivable because it's how each and every cell in the body makes energy to perform its functions. This essentially means that we CAN reverse diseases by restoring the body's ability to properly function. You'd think such a monumental study would end up in Harvard's premiere medical journal, the *New England Journal of Medicine,* but it ended up in a **science** journal instead.

We also have evidence that we can reverse aging through a similar mechanism by lengthening chromosomes. The idea that diseases should be reversed is becoming a very real possibility – this is already being explored in the fields of traditional Chinese medicine and functional medicine with natural agents, nutrition and lifestyle modifications.

What makes the Krebs Cycle go round and round...

The Krebs or citric acid cycle requires several nutrients to make energy in the body's cells. These nutrients must be obtained from the diet.

- **Macronutrients**
    - Proteins in the form of amino acids
    - Fats in the form of fatty acids
    - Carbohydrates in the form of glucose

- **Micronutrients**
    - **Vitamins**
        - Vitamin A
        - Vitamin C
        - Vitamin B1 (Thiamin)
        - Vitamin B2 (Riboflavin)
        - Vitamin B5 (Pantothenic acid)
        - Vitamin B3 (Niacin)
        - Vitamin B12 (Cobalamin)
        - Vitamin B6 (Pyridoxine)
        - Vitamin B9 (Folate)
    - **Minerals**
        - Calcium
        - Magnesium
        - Manganese

        - Zinc
        - Selenium
        - Copper
    - **Antioxidants**
        - Lipoic Acid
        - Glutathione
        - Cysteine
        - CoQ10
    - **Specific Amino Acids (found in proteins)**
        - Glutamine
        - Asparagine
        - Carnitine
        - Choline

We digest and absorb proteins, fats and carbohydrates to be used for energy production through the Krebs Cycle. Through this cycle, they're all broken down to glucose, which is a usable form of sugar. Using oxygen, one molecule of glucose yields 32 units of ATP (energy). The byproducts of energy production with oxygen are ketones, which are then burned by healthy cells; water used in cellular processes, and carbon dioxide exhaled from the lungs.

Without oxygen, one unit of glucose yields only 2 units of ATP. That's 1/16th of the amount of energy! What determines whether the cell uses oxygen to make energy or not?

- The nutrients we just listed above
- Certain lung diseases can decrease the availability of oxygen such as COPD (chronic obstructive pulmonary disease).
- Heavy metal toxins such as mercury, arsenic, antimony, and aluminum
- Fluoride, a trace mineral

Your cells may have trouble using oxygen even if your lungs are completely normal if you don't have the critical nutrients needed to complete the Krebs cycle or if there are large amounts of toxic metals that interrupt the Krebs cycle.

It's critical to be able to use adequate oxygen and have adequate nutrients so that our cells can make enough energy. A critical factor in the development of cancer cells, for example, is that cancer cells make their energy WITHOUT OXYGEN. This is called *anaerobic respiration* and is hugely important to know. When cells don't use oxygen to make energy, they produce lactic acid (see figure 10)! Lactic acid is highly toxic, and cancer cells make more pores in their cell walls to let the lactic acid out so they don't die. Our normal cells don't have this ability and are damaged by chronic lactic acid build-up. This is different than the temporary lactic acid buildup that can occur during rigorous exercise. This form of lactic acid isn't chronic and is easily eliminated by the body.

A study released in the journal *Biological Psychiatry* in 2016 linked lactic acid to **drug addiction**. Lactic acid in certain brain cells led to addiction of rodents to cocaine. These same rodents had no interest in cocaine before these cells were damaged by lactic acid. The shocking revelation was that the addicted rodents LOST their addiction to cocaine if lactic acid production was blocked! They were able to reverse addiction through the control of lactic acid production. This is monumental!

In fact, the accumulation of lactic acid due to various causes can be linked to the majority of diseases when we look from this perspective. It's critical to maintain the production of cellular energy WITH oxygen to prevent and treat diseases such as cancer, Alzheimer's dementia and even drug addiction. This also provides the opportunity to promote wellness. ***This is the unifying theory that links all diseases AND the path to their prevention!***

When the Krebs (citric acid) cycle is malfunctioning due to nutrient deficits or toxin accumulation, cells are unable to use oxygen to make energy and power body functions. This leads to self-correcting forces reshuffling resources to high-priority areas like the heart and brain and leaving lower-priority areas such as hair follicles, muscles, and even the immune system depleted.

The most critical system that keeps the Krebs cycle going round and round is the gastrointestinal system. In allopathic medicine, we are just scratching the surface to understand the complex function of the gastrointestinal system. In our conventional allopathic model, we believed the gastrointestinal system to be a continuous tube that extracts food and eliminates waste. Traditional Chinese medicine has a much more comprehensive and profound understanding through the Chinese organ system they call Spleen. We'll discuss this in the next chapter.

CHAPTER ELEVEN

GUT CHECK! (CHINESE SPLEEN)

Spleen Is King!

In TCM there's a principle that states "Spleen is King." Spleen in Chinese medicine is not what we recognize anatomically as the spleen, which lies just below the stomach in our bodies. Modern science has shown us that essentially nothing is physical, and everything is energy. The Chinese knew this thousands of years ago and we in the west began to scratch this surface about 100 years ago when Albert Einstein, my favorite historical figure next to Jesus, declared that MATTER (physical stuff) DOESN'T EXIST. He had the audacity to tell us that matter is simply energy that's so dense and vibrating so slowly that it can be detected by our rather dull senses of sight, smell, touch, taste and hearing. Of course, the scientific community wasn't thrilled with Einstein, but most of his theories have been proven true over time. He was one of the first to declare the existence of atoms and everybody thought he was crazy until science *had to admit* he was right. Today we take the existence of atoms for granted and it's no longer a debate.

When the Chinese speak of spleen, they're talking about an *energy* field that has certain functions within and *beyond* the body. We know energy fields exist within and beyond the body because we can capture them with equipment such as EKG machines, SQUIDS (superconducting quantum interference devices), Kirlian cameras, and gas discharge of photonic emissions devices. I'll discuss more about how cutting-edge modern science helps us understand and back up TCM in chapter 12. **TCM organs are energy fields**, not anatomical physical structures. All organs are interconnected and interdependent. In other words, they're like a stack of dominos. If one goes down, it takes the others with it. We can't see organs in TCM as discrete independent systems because they're not. We have labels or names for them so we can describe and understand them, but in reality, they're not separate from each other. According to TCM, spleen has 6 major functions:

1. Makes and controls blood and vital energy (called qi).
2. Governs the transformation and transportation of vital energy or qi, fluids, and food essences.
3. Controls the ascending and raising of vital energy (qi)
4. Controls the muscles and four limbs
5. Houses the intellect
6. Holds blood in the vessels

While these functions sound simplistic, they're anything but...The making of **qi (vital energy) and blood** is likely the most important body function we have. It's how we keep ourselves alive through nourishment with food. We can argue that heartbeat and breathing are more important, but *without the energy* to beat our hearts and breathe, we would die. Spleen makes this energy.

Governing transformation and transportation of vital energy and food essences is related to metabolic functions that occur in all cells of the body. The body is made of a lot of cells – somewhere on the order of 40-100 trillion; therefore, spleen affects the entire body's energy production and utilization. We can understand this through the function of the gastrointestinal system in its functions of digestion and absorption of food, AND the cells' assimilation of these nutrients and their transformation into energy in the mitochondria. Cells then use this energy in exchange for body functions such as breathing, thinking, moving, speaking, digestion, feeling joyful, reproduction, vision, hearing, hair growth, detoxification, and more.

We often think of transportation in the body as the job of the cardiovascular system: the heart propels blood rich in oxygen and nutrients through blood vessels to get to our cells. But in order to actually get *inside* our cells where the oxygen and nutrients are used, we need the transportation function of the spleen because no matter how hard the heart pumps blood through our blood vessels, it doesn't have enough force to *push* them into our cells. This requires a more subtle energy which is the responsibility of spleen – in fact, we're recognizing that transporting things *into* cells is not a physical function, but a *quantum* function. Really weird unexplainable things start to happen when we're looking on a cellular rather than grossly anatomic level. It's physically impossible for certain molecules to enter cells through our current allopathic understanding; but if we study it from a quantum physics or TCM perspective, we can begin to understand better. In fact, the emerging field of quantum biology endeavors to do just that. Quantum physics is that spooky, weird science that pioneers like Neils Bohr, Albert Einstein and Nikola Tesla forced us to look at. We use quantum physics every time we smell a flower or use our cell phones!

TCM spleen also controls the transformation and transportation of fluids in addition to qi. What does this mean? Spleen separates pure and impure fluids from what is digested in TCM spleen or the GI tract. The pure fluids ascend to the lungs where they play a role in *innate* immunity. The impure fluids go to the intestines to be further separated. If TCM spleen function isn't maintained, we accumulate what the Chinese call dampness, phlegm and edema. We understand these as different types of inflammation. Additionally, innate immunity is compromised if spleen qi is imbalanced.

Without the ascending function of spleen, our sensory organs of sight, smell, taste, hearing and touch, would be even duller or not function at all. It's through our 5 senses that we can orient ourselves in our 3D reality. We owe these functions to TCM spleen. The *raising* of qi is different than the *ascending* of qi. Raising qi has to do with keeping physical organs and structures in their correct locations. For example, when women experience a prolapsed uterus, this is the result of the failure of spleen qi to rise allowing gravity to move the uterus down into the vagina where it doesn't belong.

The TCM spleen function of housing the intellect is our ability to think, study, come up with new ideas, memorize and focus. When spleen qi is weak, we lose our ability to focus, have poor memory and concentration, and lose our creativity. If we can't focus on an experience, we can't remember it. It's through the function of spleen that we can crystalize the memory to draw upon it at a later time. Memory is very complex and is dependent on several organ systems according to TCM, the three most important of which are spleen, heart and kidney. Again, all interdependent. If one goes down, the others follow. We've recently discovered in allopathic medicine that the gastrointestinal system is the "second brain," but we haven't yet fully understood the implications. A more accurate description would be to say that the GI system and brain are interdependent. One doesn't outweigh the other in importance. The brain and nervous system are related to the TCM kidney. TCM kidney is called the "root of pre-heaven qi." It's the essence including our genes given to us by our parents at the moment of conception like a reserve tank of energy or savings account from which we spring forth. TCM spleen is called the root of "post-heaven qi." It's how we nourish ourselves after birth – akin to a checking account, so to speak. We produce energy, use it, then make more, and this goes around and around as long as spleen is functioning. If spleen function declines for any reason, we can tap into the reserve of kidney to keep going. Spleen nourishes kidney and kidney nourishes spleen. They're interdependent.

In allopathic conventional medicine, we understand the GI system to be a tube that runs from our mouth to our anus assimilating food and eliminating waste. So, we've essentially understood part of the function of TCM spleen, but we haven't even begun to understand the other functions as assigned by TCM, but we are starting to scratch the surface.

The Gut Ecosystem

The Human Genome Project was completed in 2005 to study the human genetic code. Given how complex the physiology of the human body is, we expected to find a lot to pat ourselves on the back about when we undertook this monumental endeavor. We expected to find millions of genes in the DNA of our cells to explain our complexity, but we were disappointed to find that we have about as many genes as a common houseplant: 25,000 functional genes. If we add the so-called "non-functional" genes, the number rises to 48,000 – still rather disappointing.

In 2012, the U.S. government undertook the Human MICROBIOME Project to study the genetic code of the 100,000,000,000,000 (yes, 100 trillion) bugs that inhabit our lower gastrointestinal tract. We call them the microbiome. These bacteria are part of the human body. What we found was nearly incomprehensible. The Human Microbiome Project was a humbling experience – the bugs we've taken for granted and systematically tried to destroy for the last century through the use of pesticides and antibiotics house 3,400,000 (3.4 million) genes that we need to live. We literally can't live without them! In fact, we owe our ability to be human to bacteria. The mitochondria which produce energy in multicellular organisms like us are descendants of bacteria! We acquire these bugs at birth while passing through the birth canal. A study released in September 2019 at the University of London showed that babies born by cesarean section are colonized by different bacteria than babies born by vaginal birth. The babies born by cesarean section had pathogenic bacteria, which are potentially infectious microbes. Babies born by vaginal delivery had normal microbiome flora. This study suggests what's been suspected for some time: vaginal delivery protects babies and provides improved immunity.

The microbiome through its 3.4 million genes affects blood sugar control, cholesterol, amino acid (protein) metabolism, cellular energy production, detoxification, and vitamin synthesis. These bugs regulate immunity, prevent overgrowth of dangerous bacteria, and regulate bowel movements. The notion that *spleen* is responsible for keeping blood in the blood vessels is also explained in this way: Those little bugs help make vitamin K, which is involved in blood clotting. Low levels of vitamin K are associated with bleeding disorders and easy bruising. Modern medicine hasn't completely explained all the functions that the Chinese have given this marvelous organ system called spleen, but we can confidently use Chinese medicine to treat today's problems.

Keeping the Chinese spleen and gut healthy is responsible for treating depression and other mental health disorders. Taking probiotics, which increase the numbers of commensal bacteria that belong in the gut, has been shown to help depression and even bipolar disorder in recent studies. There's emerging controversy about how to rebalance the microbiome when it loses balance, and the evidence to support the long-term use of probiotics is lacking, however, the use of *pre*biotics is emerging as a more viable option. Prebiotics are not bugs, but rather types of carbohydrates called fructo-oligosaccharides and galacto-oligosaccharides, that are not digested by the human gastrointestinal system but instead are eaten by the bugs of the microbiome serving as a kind of fertilizer for their growth. Studies are showing that this may be a safer way to support the microbiome long-term.

There's also ample medical evidence for the use of TCM herbal therapies for support and modulation of the microbiome. Herbs such as gan cao (licorice root) and huang qin (skullcap root) have been shown to have important effects on the microbiome. Again, a doctor certified to use these modalities should prescribe Chinese herbs after careful evaluation. The support of the microbiome is paramount to wellness and has been shown to help treat diabetes, cancer, Alzheimer's dementia and more. We'll see why in the next section.

A 1998 article published in the journal *Microbiology and Molecular Biology Review* revealed the following: "The relationship between a human host and its intestinal commensal bacterial flora is to a large extent symbiotic." In other words, we need the bugs as much as they need us. There's that interdependence principle again. All mammals, including humans, are adapted to life in a microbial world. The scientists Pasteur, Koch, Metchnikoff, and Escherich laid the conceptual groundwork for our present views of host-microbe interactions. Pasteur postulated that microbes are necessary for normal human life. Metchnikoff claimed that the composition of the flora is essential for the well-being of the host and stressed the importance of interactions between host and bacteria. Escherich was convinced that accurate knowledge of this flora was essential not only for understanding the physiology of digestion but also for understanding the pathology and therapy of microbial intestinal diseases. Despite these early insights, scientists have only recently developed methods that allow them to directly characterize the molecular mechanisms underlying the establishment and maintenance of various microbial ecosystems located on or in the human body. The journal *Microbiology and Molecular Biology Review* further states that the gastrointestinal ecosystem or microbiome also modulates the lymphatic system located in the gut. The gastrointestinal tract contains more immune cells than the rest of the body. Lymphoid cells such as B cells and T cells are a critical part of the body's immune system. The gut houses more of these lymphoid cells than the lymphatics system, anatomical spleen, and blood combined! 80% of the entire body's B cells lives in the gastrointestinal system. Another critical component of the immune system, the T-lymphocytes are also housed in the gastrointestinal tract! **T cells and B cells are the main immune cells responsible for killing cancer cells**. Because the gastrointestinal tract houses a huge portion of lymphocytes or immune cells, there's a delicate balance between the commensal bacteria and these immune cells. When the bacterial ecosystem is out of balance, the immune system can't properly function. This increases the risk of diseases, not just of the gastrointestinal tract but systemic diseases like autoimmune disease, depression, anxiety, heart disease, Alzheimer dementia, and even autism.

Given all this data, it's no surprise that antibiotics, which kill the bacteria of the microbiome, are linked to escalating new cases of certain cancers. Another point to make here is that most antibiotics are synthetic and artificial, which poses a challenge for the body to eliminate. So, the perfect storm begins to form: We have a weak immune system from chronic stress and antibiotics in addition to a load of toxins. This all leads to diseases like Alzheimer's dementia, heart disease, cancer and more. There are more natural and effective alternatives than antibiotics that can kill and suppress pathological bacteria ***while sparing the commensal bacteria***. Knowledge is power. A study conducted by Johns Hopkins University in 2014 showed that *herbal formulas were as effective or better than an antibiotic* called Rifaximin for small intestine bacterial overgrowth, a significant infection of the small intestine that can be debilitating for many people. Moving towards safer options for infections will be a critical step in restoring proper body function.

Current State of the American Gut

The load of toxins and poor quality of the food that we eat set us up for many diseases, but what has likely been the most damaging to the GI system is the injudicious use of antibiotics and use of pesticides. Antibiotics are a major cause of many gastrointestinal concerns, but more importantly, they lead to systemic diseases **outside** of the gastrointestinal system.

Antibiotics can be indirectly responsible for sleep disorders, depression, arthritis, heart disease, Alzheimer's dementia, and even cancer, just to name a few. This is because of their impact on the gut. The gut is a very delicate system that is self-maintained and corrected, but it has its limits. Antibiotics wipe out a variety of normally needed bacteria in the gastrointestinal tract, on your skin, and in other areas of the body. These bacteria are part of the human body and perform critical functions that are lost after taking antibiotics. Many people don't suffer gastrointestinal symptoms after using antibiotics and don't realize they're damaging their guts and immune systems (or TCM *spleen*) until much later.

What Happens When the Gut Doesn't Work?

When the gut or Chinese *spleen* doesn't work properly due to damage, disease, or energy imbalances, many conditions can arise: hernias, prolapsed uterus, urinary incontinence, easy bruising, varicose veins, abnormal menstrual bleeding, diarrhea, constipation, bloating, fatigue, sleep disturbances, malabsorption, depression, other psychiatric diseases, and even cancer. Weak immunity, such as frequent colds or allergies, can all be caused by gut dysfunction or *spleen* deficiency. Even weight gain can be caused by gut dysfunction.

How To Evaluate and Treat the Gut

Allopathic medicine evaluates the gut if there are significant intestinal symptoms, such as pain, diarrhea, or change in bowel habits. Screening for colon cancer usually begins at age 50 for most low-risk people. Significant gastrointestinal symptoms may trigger a colonoscopy or an endoscopy, which is looking at the surface of the gastrointestinal tract. These procedures look for anatomically visible conditions, such as gastritis, polyps, colon cancer, and diverticulosis.

Frequently not much is found during these evaluations to explain symptoms. This is because these procedures are looking for anatomical changes which are very late presentations of problems that occur once disease has taken hold. There is essentially no testing available in allopathic medicine to look into the *function* of the gastrointestinal system.

A TCM evaluation of the gut almost always leads to answers that can be further explored or treated. TCM determines patterns of disharmony or imbalance that take the entire body and its environment into consideration. Answers can almost always be found using a TCM examination. For thousands of years, acupuncture and traditional Chinese herbal therapy have been shown to be very effective in treating many gut conditions. Although not part of TCM, functional testing can also be used to target the root cause of the condition long before diseases take hold; and even if diseases are present, the root causes can begin to be treated so that the disease can be successfully treated.

Looking at the surface of the gut, such as with allopathic medicine, leads to late diagnosis of problems that can be corrected at a much earlier stage if more holistic evaluation principles are used. It's very important to diagnose colon cancer; however, it's much more important to *prevent* it. We can perform a biopsy during endoscopy or colonoscopy, but it's almost impossible to know where to biopsy unless it's obvious, and even then, only certain conditions can be diagnosed once they've taken hold. That's not prevention. Prevention requires looking at the gut differently from an energetic or functional perspective. How can we evaluate below the surface to find this information? With cellular-based functional gut testing, a whole new world is visible that can help prevent diseases and repair damage. Stool samples are often used in allopathic medicine to diagnose certain kinds of infections, such as bacterial, fungal, or parasitic infection in the stool, but so much more can be determined from this that can help heal the gut and ultimately the entire body since it's one connected whole.

Using functional medicine, stool samples and breath testing can be used to give so much more information. What will likely be recognized as an epidemic infection is an infection known as SIBO or small intestine bacterial overgrowth. It's currently not recognized by most mainstream allopathic physicians although it's been studied by respected institutions such as Johns Hopkins and Yale Universities. This insidious quiet infection can be present for years and never diagnosed because it's not seen on any X-ray, CT, MRI or endoscopy studies. The danger of this infection is not that it causes any gastrointestinal symptoms, although it can cause belching, diarrhea, constipation, bloating and more. The real danger is that it prevents absorption of critical nutrients needed for body function throughout the body. SIBO is being recognized as an underlying contributing factor to many diseases such as cancer, Alzheimer dementia, diabetes, and more. It must be diagnosed through a breath test that detects gases emitted by these bugs that are well hidden in the small intestine. Treating this infection can be tricky because it's not possible at this time to identify the bugs responsible without fairly invasive procedures, which are usually reserved for clinical studies. Even more critical is that antibiotics have not been shown to be more effective than herbal therapies to date. Having this infection identified by a board-certified integrative medical doctor and properly treated is of paramount importance in any wellness plan.

Through the use of functional stool sampling, the members of the microbiome can be identified, their numbers and metabolic functions estimated to help you know if you need probiotic or prebiotic support. You can know if you need digestive enzymes to help break down your food for digestion and absorption, as opposed to just guessing. You can also know if you have inflammation and need further testing for food intolerances. Food intolerances are caused by gastrointestinal disturbances that disrupt immune system function leading to exaggerated responses by your cells when exposed to certain foods. They're not the same as food allergies. Food intolerances exacerbate the already existing inflammation in your body and can lead to disease.

You can also tell if you have poor absorption of foods, as absorption markers are tested using stool and urine samples in functional medicine. There's so much you can learn and correct to help prevent diseases, but this information isn't available at your conventional allopathic doctor's office. And sadly, many patients who approach their conventional allopathic doctors for help with these issues are ridiculed for suggesting that a more holistic and natural route be taken for diagnosis and treatment.

How To Bypass the Gut If It's Not Working

Some people have such significant gut problems that taking even the best oral supplements to correct them don't work because the very system that absorbs them into the body isn't working. Then what? Sounds like a catch-22, doesn't it?

Nutrients can be used intravenously and placed directly into the bloodstream to go directly to the body's cells to help with healing. This is a safe and practical way to still get nutrition, even if the gut isn't working properly.

In allopathic medicine, we sometimes use IV nutrients when patients are hospitalized and can't eat for extended periods of time. In integrative medicine, we can also use IV nutrition in a much more comprehensive and practical way as an outpatient or even at home, if malabsorption is present or when patients are simply not getting better with oral therapies. The highest quality oral supplements have an average of 30% absorption due to the gastrointestinal tract and what's known as first-pass metabolism through the liver. Since the liver is a detoxification organ, it eliminates the additional vitamins and minerals found in supplements, leaving only 30% available to the body's cells. IV nutrition bypasses both the gut and liver and allows 100% of the nutrients to reach the cells. IV nutrition allows the body to get nutrition and also helps the gut to heal because it's not in its own way.

While undergoing an IV therapy program, healing strategies help the gut get better so that you can use oral supplements and food over time. It's absolutely critical to heal any gut issues before they get more serious, not just to prevent gut diseases such as colon cancer, but to prevent all kinds of other diseases indirectly related, like other forms of cancer, Alzheimer dementia, autoimmune disorders, heart disease and more.

Yes, fixing your abdominal bloating today can prevent cancer later and heart disease, too. Healing your gut can save your life! My client, whom I'll call Debbie to mask her identity, came to me just after a diagnosis of breast cancer. She had a history of severe fibrocystic disease despite living a healthy lifestyle of good nutrition and exercise. Debbie came to see me due to hot flashes and night sweats that kept her up at night. She also had abdominal bloating and occasional loose stools as minor symptoms. What drove her to seek care was that her hot flashes were disturbing her sleep. My TCM-based assessment of Debbie revealed *liver-spleen* disharmony with toxic heat and stasis.

Loosely translated, this meant that Debbie's liver was not detoxifying properly and she was building up acidity leading to poor circulation, and her gastrointestinal system and metabolism were weak. Additionally, her TCM kidney qi was weak, and she was likely missing hormone and nutrient support. Based on this, I prescribed acupuncture to "course" the liver, invigorate blood, and clear heat, which helped her symptoms. I also prescribed an alkaline diet for Debbie to help reduce overacidity and eliminate toxins.

Cellular-based testing revealed adrenal fatigue (see chapter 13) and estrogen dominance. Estrogen dominance is known to cause excessive growth of breast cells. Her nutrient analysis revealed deficiency in vitamins B12, pantothenic acid (also a B vitamin), copper, zinc, selenium, manganese, vitamin D3, and lipoic acid. Debbie had a perfect storm in her body for the diagnosis of breast cancer. Adrenal fatigue and many of the nutrients in which she was deficient are known as breast cancer risk factors.

Debbie's symptoms didn't improve with the oral nutrient therapy. The acupuncture, which didn't rely on her gut function, worked well. I proceeded with functional testing of her gastrointestinal system and found the following: small intestine bacterial overgrowth, fat and protein malabsorption, low microbiome diversity, microbiome metabolic disturbance, and leaky gut. I prescribed digestive enzymes, herbal treatment to eradicate the small bowel infection, and probiotics. I subsequently treated her leaky gut with specific supplements.

Remember, the only gut symptom Debbie had was a little bloating and occasional loose stools, and this was just the tip of a very large iceberg that was making her very sick. Debbie is well on her way to being as healthy as she's ever been despite a significant setback. Debbie had an uncomplicated treatment of her breast cancer consisting of removal of the cancerous lump. She declined chemotherapy and radiation therapy and used more natural methods with great success. She's been cancer-free for several years and she continues to keep a watchful eye on the underlying causes of cancer. When we use the principles of TCM combined with cellular-based testing as found in functional medicine, we can remain focused on the root causes and successfully resolve them even when a serious disease is already present. In the next chapter, I'll discuss how modern cutting-edge science is confirming the principles of TCM and functional medicine. It turns out that the truth is hidden in plain sight…if we choose to look.

CHAPTER TWELVE

THE CUTTING EDGE OF THE CUTTING EDGE:

How Modern Science Backs Up TCM And Energy Based Principles

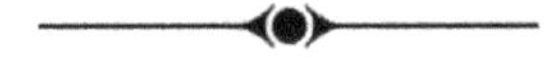

$E = mc^2$ is arguably the most famous scientific equation of all time. In simple terms, this equation states that energy and matter (physical things) are essentially the same. Energy can become physical things and physical things can become energy. Albert Einstein shockingly stated that matter, in fact, doesn't even exist and is simply energy that's vibrating so slowly that it's perceived by our limited senses as matter or a physical thing.

Albert Einstein opened up a can of worms with his famous equation that became part of a revolution in science: quantum physics. He didn't perform any scientific experiments to determine his theory. It just came to him; then it was applied and **proven true later**. TCM is based in quantum physics and energy, and is over 4,000 years old. Ancient wisdom and medical traditions blend perfectly with modern science when we look at the relationship from the correct perspective.

A growing body of scientific evidence over the past decade is suggesting that several biological systems use quantum physics. For example, the process of photosynthesis, how plants make their energy, appears to involve quantum effects to turn sunlight into fuel. Migratory birds appear to use quantum effects to use the earth's electromagnetic field for navigation. Even the human sense of smell is now being considered as a possible quantum effect. In TCM, the body itself is considered a quantum energy field and the organs that they describe are energy fields, not physical structures.

Although few people on earth understand quantum physics, we use it every day in cell phone technology as energy waves carry conversations through space. We prove quantum physics to ourselves every time we use our cell phones or smell a rose. The launching of satellites into space involves quantum physics. We're developing quantum computers to help us compute things we could never tackle with ordinary computers.

Thanks to pioneers like Albert Einstein and Neils Bohr, quantum physics is teaching modern man that *energy happens before matter "forms."* And further, matter is just really dense energy!

"Concerning matter, we have been all wrong.
What we have called matter is energy,
whose vibration has been so lowered
as to be perceptible to the senses.
There is no matter."

--Albert Einstein

"There is no matter." Wow. Einstein made this shocking statement that is now being accepted by quantum physicists, although *allopathic medicine has not yet come to this realization.*

Every "thing," or what we call matter, is energy first in the form of a wave that collapses or drops so low in frequency that it can be perceived by our senses as a thing like a wall, a cloud, a planet, a body, or any other "thing" we can think of. Knowing this about energy is critical to our well-being. Allopathic medicine ignores this fact and this is one of the main reasons it's failed to keep the American population healthy. Allopathic medicine is based on physical structures such as organs and chemicals, and ignores the fact that it's all really just energy and part of a much larger energy field. If we can't detect it with our "medical devices" or prove it with our outdated modes of experimentation, then we don't believe it to be real and this has been a significant downfall of Allopathic medicine.

Allopathic medicine ignores the fundamental idea that balancing energy allows the physical matter of the body to heal; but one monumental and "unadvertised" medical study that was released in the journal *Cell* in March 2019 may begin to reverse this trajectory. Scientists at the Massachusetts Institute of Technology were able to dissolve Alzheimer's-associated amyloid plaques in mice using light and sound energy! In essence, what these scientists were able to achieve was to alter the vibration of the cells and atoms leading to a reorganization and normalization of the "matter" in the brain using frequencies of light and sound energy. Of course, this mind-blowing study received no attention and went unnoticed by most of the scientific and medical community, so we still have a long way to go before allopathic medicine embraces this concept, but this is an exciting start!

Chinese medicine is an energy-based system of medicine that uses the balancing of energy as its main focus to balance the body and its functions. Knowing that matter is really just dense and slow vibrating energy helps us understand why TCM can work as well as it has for thousands of years.

Quantum physics further suggests that what we perceive as matter is really just energy with forces acting on it, making it "feel like" matter or physical substance. In fact, at the time of the big bag, which is widely agreed to be how this Universe exploded into existence, all of the matter we currently have in our universe was squeezed down into the size of a *grain of sand.* Some theoretical physicists such as Nasim Haramein suggest that the universe was actually born out a singularity, which is infinitely smaller than a grain of sand. **This implies very strongly that everything we see or sense today was at one time connected to everything else we see or sense because it all originated from a common source**. Take a moment to sit with that last sentence. It's critically important to our understanding of our oneness. In fact, what we're beginning to realize is that everything we see and sense in our universe today is **still** connected to everything else in the universe despite vast distances between them. MIT, the Max Planck Institute, and Harvard University have collaborated on a project which suggests that **the entire universe is, in fact, connected as energy.** TCM theory is based on the body being one connected whole while being intimately connected with the environment as well. One energy field. In TCM, everything is one...mind, body, spirit...all one. From these foundational perspectives, we can see the relationship between quantum physics and TCM theory begin to unfold.

A shocking experiment done in quantum physics was the "double slit experiment" which has been reproduced in multiple other labs throughout the world. This classic experiment showed that light or photons, which are fundamental building blocks of the universe are *both* waves of energy *and* particles of matter.

What determines if the photon behaves like energy or collapses into matter is actually determined by whether there is an "observer" of the photon. This approximates what we're now beginning to understand as *consciousness*. If there is an "observer" or consciousness focusing on this energy, the light picks ***one*** *of two slits as though it were a particle of physical matter*. But if we take the "observer" or consciousness away, the photon acts like a wave of energy and goes through ***both*** *slits at the same time like a wave*. So, the **energy is present first and collapses into matter once something focuses on it to make it so**. (See figure 11.)

This implies that when we harness this energy with our focus *before* it exists as a physical *thing*, we're pulling it out of infinite quantum possibility and transforming it into our linear physical reality as matter or physical substances. This makes focused intention and energy pretty important for healing the body and mind. The human body is a field of energy vibrating slowly enough that it can be perceived as a physical thing. When we perceive a symptom or disease, this is a sign of energy imbalance. Rebalancing the energy can heal this energy field leading to healing of the physical body on a cellular level, as well as the mind.

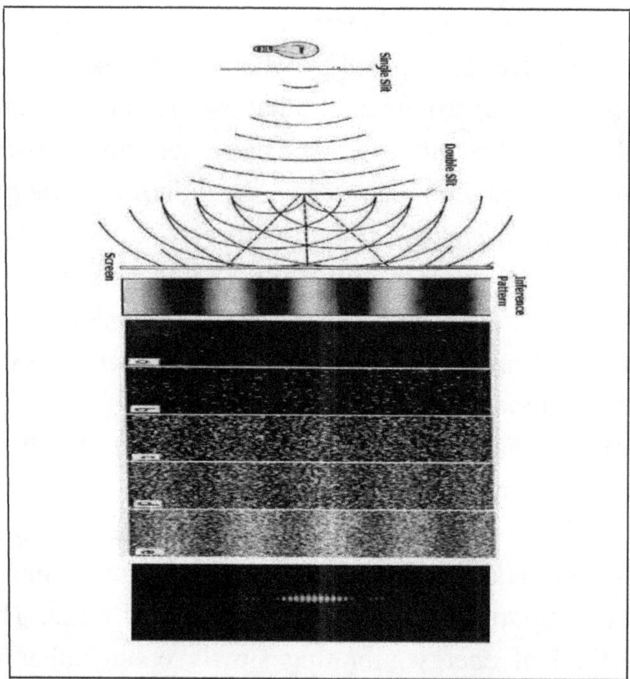

Figure 11: The classic double-slit experiment demonstrates that a photon of light is both a wave and a particle. As a photon from a light passes through two parallel slits, it results in an interference pattern producing light and dark bands on the screen, demonstrating the wave-like properties of the photons of light. However, on the screen are found discrete points or particles. The interference pattern is formed by the density of these particles hitting the screen. Where there are more particles on the screen, we see a light band and where there are fewer particles on the screen, we see a dark band. A startling observation is made when a detector is placed at the two slits through which the photon passes. Each photon of light passes through only one slit and not both, as would be expected if light were a wave.

In addition to that little equation, $E = mc^2$, Albert Einstein also predicted the existence of atoms before any other scientist, and he was widely ridiculed for this idea. Today, nobody doubts thc existence of atoms. Albert Einstein was decades ahead of his time! He actually discovered another profound principle, but found it so strange, he called it "spooky action at a distance." At the time, this principle defied the science that we understood in the West. Einstein was convinced that there must be some other "reality" that would explain this principle, but he couldn't figure it out prior to his death. We now use the term *quantum entanglement* to describe what Einstein called "spooky action at a distance."

"Spooky action at a distance" says that if we alter a particle in the universe, this *instantaneously* affects its "twin" particle no matter where that particle is located in the universe. In other words, the particles are instantly communicating beyond what is possible in the known universe - not just faster than the speed of light, but with *absolutely no passage of time*. It's considered impossible for anything *inside* the universe to travel faster than the speed of light. So, this implies that this interaction is happening *outside* the known universe.

Since then scientists have been debating whether or not this principle could be true - that particles on the opposite ends of the universe could be entangled, in other words, ***connected OUTSIDE of space and time*, in some other undiscovered reality**. An experiment in the Netherlands, published by *Nature International Journal of Science* in October 2015, showed that spooky action at a distance, or quantum entanglement, is real! Other similar experiments have been recently conducted showing the same results.

What's important to see here is that the particles aren't traveling so fast in physical reality that they're going faster than the speed of light. They're not influencing each other inside the universe at all. They act independently of each other but are entangled at the same time, which is why this is such a mind-blowing concept. This is where the notion of a collective consciousness is taking root in scientific terms. We can see this as individuals. We are each independent beings, but also entangled with each other at the same time. We have our individual consciousness and our collective consciousness. What each of us does independently affects the collective as a whole. This makes the golden rule that much more important, doesn't it? ***It also appears***

that the "reality" where entanglement exists is a foundational necessity for the existence of the universe itself. Without this other reality, we cannot exist.

I found a great example of the notion of entanglement in a magazine called Science News. The author, Tom Siegfried, gives the following example: Alice is in one city and is mailed a single glove. She gets the glove and sees that it's a right-handed glove. So, she can assume that if her friend Bob, who lives in a different city, also received a single glove as part of this pair, that his would be left-handed. *BUT quantum entanglement is not that simple.* Quantum entanglement is as if Alice was mailed a *mitten* and when she opened the box and put the mitten on her right hand, it *became* a right-handed *glove*. Bob also got a mitten in the mail, but his mitten only became a glove *if* he placed it on his left hand! If Bob placed the mitten on his right hand (the hand that Alice had previously placed her mitten on), it would remain a mitten, and never become a glove because the two mittens are entangled so it can only become a glove if Bob places it on his left hand. This is what experiments are showing us about quantum entanglement and the *other reality* we're just discovering with science.

In ancient traditions, the idea of a collective consciousness has been known for millennia and isn't even questioned. It appears that science is inching its way towards the same conclusion as it follows the evidence left by quantum entanglement and other principles of quantum physics.

I'm not a quantum physicist and my understanding of this mind-blowing science is quite limited, but I'll share with you here what I know. Quantum physics is based on the theory that particles of matter are waves of energy, and waves of energy are particles of matter. In other words, energy and matter are essentially the same things with different vibrations. Frequency is the speed at which a wave of energy vibrates. Certain forms of energy vibrate so fast that we can't perceive them. For example, dogs can hear sound with a frequency as high as 60,000 Hz (cycles per second). Humans generally can't hear anything higher than 20,000 Hz. Just because we can't perceive this energy doesn't mean it doesn't exist. Matter is simply energy that is vibrating at such a low frequency, we can sense it with our eyes, ears, noses, touch, or with certain instruments.

Quantum physics is also based on the idea that the position *and* momentum of a particle can never *both* be known. In other words, until the wave transforms or collapses into a particle of matter or physical thing, *it doesn't actually exist in the physical world*, but is in an *infinite pool of possible* energies. $E = mc^2$.

Quantum physics is that science that shows that the earth is round rather than flat as we move away from the earth. Classical or Newtonian physics leads us to believe that the earth is flat because, as we sit on the earth and look out on the horizon, it looks flat. These are observable properties on earth due to the relative slow speed and large size from which we view it. Standing on the earth you would never know that it's spinning at 18,000 miles per hour around its axis! But if you go into outer space, you quickly realize that the Earth is moving at breakneck speed! The earth exerts a gravitational pull that causes the apple to fall towards the earth rather than just float in space. If you move away from the earth into outer space, that same apple will not fall to the ground, but will instead float in space.

In space we can definitely see that the earth is definitely round and NOT flat. Because the earth is relatively smaller as viewed from outer space, we can use our instruments such as our eyes to clearly see that it's round. On the earth, our eyes are viewing the earth as *relatively* much larger, so our eyes are limited and we falsely think it's flat. This is the difference between quantum physics and classical Newtonian physics. Classical Newtonian physics is active at relative low speed and large size, such as on earth. Quantum physics is active at relative high speed and small size such as far in outer space… or ***deep in our cells***.

Our ability to measure things that are very large is limited by the precision of the tools we use to measure them. Our eyes are quite limited, so as we look on the horizon as we sit on the earth, our eyes fail to see the curvature in the earth and it looks flat.

When things get immeasurably small such as at a quantum or atomic level, our ability to measure is equally poor, and things become uncertain and immeasurable. We can't tell where an electron is in an atom with precision. We can only state a probability that the electron may be in a certain position within the atom.

Inside our cells, things become immeasurably small and are influenced by the laws of *quantum* physics much more so than *Newtonian* physics. So, on a macroscopic level the body as an anatomical machine appears to behave according to Newtonian physics. If you jump up in the air, gravity will bring you back down. On a microscopic level, when things become immeasurably small, such as in our cells, the body behaves more according to quantum physics. A growing body of scientific evidence over the past decade is suggesting that several biological systems use quantum physics. For example, the process of photosynthesis which turns sunlight into fuel in plants is now thought to be a quantum phenomenon. Migratory birds appear to use quantum effects to use the earth's electromagnetic field for navigation. Even the human sense of smell is now being considered as a possible quantum effect. As scientists investigate the inside of human cells, it appears that quantum physics is busy at work.

Allopathic medicine uses principles of Newtonian physics almost exclusively, rather than using both, and this limits what it can describe and treat. If we can't see or detect it with our eyes or blood work, x-rays, etc…then we falsely believe that nothing is there. *This is what leads allopathic physicians to tell patients that everything is normal, when it's not.*

The mind-blowing continues with a computer simulation of the universe called the Illustris Project, done through the collaboration between the Massachusetts Institute of Technology (MIT), Harvard University, the Heidelberg Institute, and the Max Planck Institute. It's long been known that what we see when we look up into the sky is only a fraction of what's out there. In fact, the physical matter we saw in the universe even with our strongest telescopes only made up less than 4% of the Universe, and we knew for a long time that there was a huge chunk of the universe that we couldn't yet detect. We called these dark matter and dark energy, not yet understanding what they even were. The Illustris scientists used **x-ray** telescopes such as the NASA Chandra telescope. Typically, we use **optical** telescopes which look at physical structures like stars, galaxies, and planets by using light to reflect off the objects. The Chandra x-ray telescope is different. It's an energy telescope that detects energy in the x-ray spectrum, which is electromagnetic radiation. X-ray telescopes are 100 million times more sensitive than an optical telescope. They used these images and the known laws of the universe to simulate a 3-D model of the universe from just after the big bang to the present, and the results have been shocking! When you look at the "invisible" or dark universe, everything is connected like a spider web, and the physicists refer to this as the "cosmic web." (See figure 12).

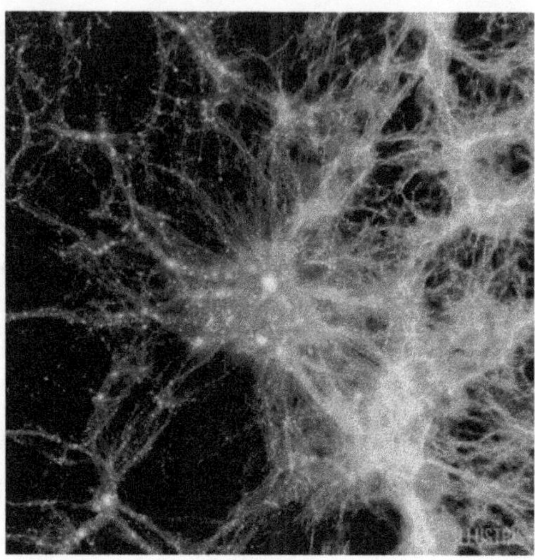

Figure 12: The "Cosmic Web." Credit: The Illustris Collaboration / Illustris Simulation

---

Where the bright regions appear in the cosmic web is where galaxies are located. It appears that since the entire universe started condensed into the size smaller than a pea, *everything was originally connected and* ***remains connected*** *despite the vast distances between them.* You can follow the story at http://www.tng-project.org. The original project called Illustris can be viewed at http://www.illustris-project.org. The idea that the universe is a connected whole has monumental implications as it also implies that *we are all connected and therefore, interdependent*. What we put out in the universe affects others and returns to us because we're all connected!

When you look at the universe from an anatomical "physical matter" perspective, all you see are the stars, planets and other celestial bodies as seen in figure 13. The energetic connections are not visible with an optical telescope which leads us to mistakenly believe they are separate. The bright regions in figure 13 would correspond with the bright regions in the Illustris image of figure 12 above, which are galaxies.

Chinese medicine understood these energetic principles of quantum physics thousands of years ago despite not having access to today's technology, and TCM still works today just as it did then. It's fundamental and universal. It's based on the fact that the human body is an organic and whole energetic entity, intimately connected to its environment on all levels just as scientists are showing the Universe is connected through the cosmic web.

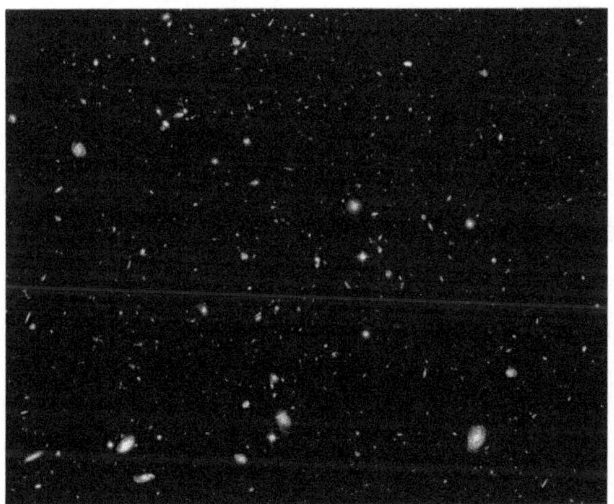

Figure 13: ESA/Hubble Image called "Hubble Sees Galaxies Galore." This starting image actually contains nearly 10,000 galaxies and is the deepest visible-light view of the cosmos.

We're emitting electromagnetic fields and charges as discovered at the Institute of HeartMath®, and are constantly interacting and changing with the environment through these electromagnetic fields or energies; just as modern physicists have discovered about many other biological systems.

In fact, scientists are now determining that the Great Pyramid at Giza in Egypt can focus electromagnetic energy from the Earth into its internal chambers as well as in the chamber under its base. This study was conducted by international scientists using theoretical physics principles and their findings were published in the *Journal of Applied Physics* in July 2018 – again, without fanfare. This study implies that the Great Pyramid was not simply a burial chamber as commonly believed, but may have been a place of healing. Energy based medicine has roots that stretch back thousands of years through multiple cultures.

Chinese medicine excels at diagnosing the underlying root causes and imbalances in energy that cause symptoms and diseases. Our allopathic system simply can't do this, which is why it's becoming obsolete for today's complex chronic medical conditions and, this is why we've become much sicker under its watch. Chinese medicine also excels at the maintenance of wellness as it can see energy imbalances long before they become symptoms - another property that our allopathic medical system simply doesn't have.

In the next chapter, I'll use the principles we've discussed so far to demystify some medical controversies, that when properly understood, are not controversial at all.

CHAPTER THIRTEEN

MEDICAL CONTROVERSIES DEMYSTIFIED

In this chapter, I'll address some "controversies" caused by misinformation and confusion. Once we begin to look at these controversies logically, we see that there really aren't any controversies at all, just misinformation. Certain medical topics have been needlessly mired in controversy for decades. The specific systems and conditions I'll address here are the adrenal glands, liver, thyroid, gastrointestinal system, and hormones which are part of the endocrine system. Vitamins are so controversial that they have their own chapter.

Adrenal Fatigue: Real or Imagined?

The adrenal glands are tiny glands located above the anatomical kidneys. They're responsible for the fight-or-flight mechanisms of the body. It's largely believed in allopathic medicine that these glands are always working normally except in rare circumstances. Addison's disease, or adrenal insufficiency, is an extremely rare condition in which the adrenal glands can't sufficiently respond to stressors to the point of being life threatening. The body can't maintain blood pressure and heart rate so patients must be maintained with medications called corticosteroids. People who suffer from Addison's are tired, dizzy, and are so incapable of responding to stress that it can kill them.

Looking for A Needle in A Haystack — Addison's Disease

Addison's disease is a fringe disease that affects less than one percent of the population. John Fitzgerald Kennedy, our former President, had Addison's disease. This condition is diagnosed through bloodwork using a stimulant to measure the response of the adrenal glands. If cortisol levels are below normal in bloodwork, this is diagnostic of Addison's.

The problem is that many patients have significant fatigue, low blood pressure, dizziness, infertility, and erectile dysfunction but don't meet criteria for Addison's disease with bloodwork, but they do have an adrenal condition that remains undiagnosed. The allopathic medical community doesn't recognize that there are stages of adrenal disorders that occur prior to the diagnosis of Addison's disease. As conventional allopathically-trained medical doctors, we're trained to understand that the adrenal glands are always working perfectly unless you have Addison's disease or another condition called Cushing's disease. There's no consideration that there's a spectrum that leads to Addison's disease, and because Addison's is so rare, there's no focus on the assessment of this critical system. Part of the reason for this is that the *disorders that precede Addison's cann't be diagnosed with blood work*. You must look inside the cells to see these stages, and because blood work remains the "gold standard" in conventional allopathic medicine, we miss the boat. This leads many physicians to conclude that the adrenals are working fine, when they aren't. The reason it's so difficult to find an adrenal disorder with bloodwork goes back to the fact that your body knows better. It's well aware that it has to maintain cortisol in the bloodstream so that it reaches those critical systems that are responsible for fight-or-flight — our brain, heart, and our lungs — so it maintains normal blood levels of cortisol in order to assure survival. Here are those self-correcting forces at work again. It stands to reason that the adrenals wouldn't go from stone-cold normal to Addison's disease. There has to be a spectrum in between.

When we have symptoms of a weakened adrenal system, called adrenal fatigue in integrative medicine, and we look in the bloodstream for causes, we won't find any answers. This is why saliva testing is being increasingly proven to be more valuable and is becoming the gold standard for the diagnosis of many adrenal conditions, such as adrenal fatigue or stress. Even allopathic medical journals are recognizing that cellular levels of cortisol are more sensitive than blood levels.

The adrenal glands are much more important than they're given credit for. They're the root of the body; they wake up all your organs when you get up every morning. They also respond with a fight-or-flight response when the body is under stress. If we're exposed to a life-threatening predator, the adrenal glands, or the system that initiates the fight-or-flight response, instantaneously raises blood pressure and heart rate; sugar is pumped into our bloodstream to get our muscles ready to fight or run. With adrenal fatigue, these responses don't occur properly and go undiagnosed with bloodwork. Since we're not often exposed to life-threatening predators in our modern era, this lack of response expresses instead as fatigue, low blood pressure, dizziness, possible weight gain, increased susceptibility to infections, and low or unstable blood sugar.

The Survival Instinct When We're Near the Top of the Food Chain

As I've stressed throughout this book, the fight-or-flight mechanism is critical for survival and hasn't changed over time as we've moved up on the food chain over the past 200,000 years. You might say that's a good thing, but wait, nobody sent our cells the memo that we've neared the top of the food chain. Cells don't have brains or eyes and can't read memos. Your cells rely on chemicals called hormones to enter them and tell them what to do.

Adrenal hormones are principally responsible for the fight-or-flight response. The acute fight-or-flight response is mediated by the adrenal hormones epinephrine and norepinephrine. Once the acute phase is over, which lasts a few minutes, cortisol is released until the threat is perceived to be gone. (See Figure 14.)

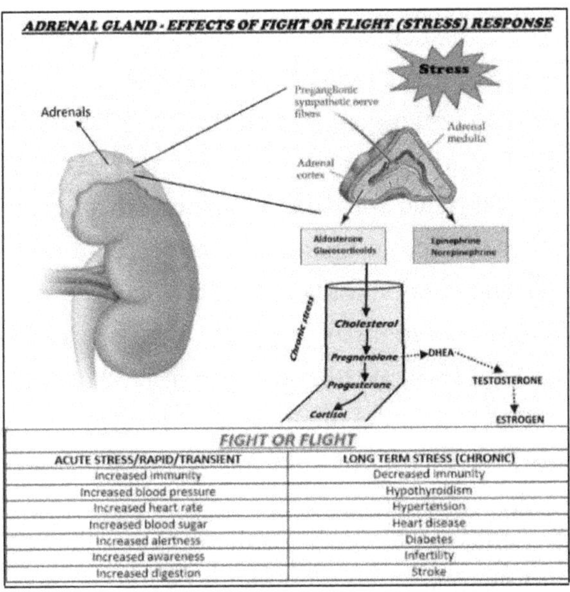

FIGHT OR FLIGHT	
ACUTE STRESS/RAPID/TRANSIENT	LONG TERM STRESS (CHRONIC)
Increased immunity	Decreased immunity
Increased blood pressure	Hypothyroidism
Increased heart rate	Hypertension
Increased blood sugar	Heart disease
Increased alertness	Diabetes
Increased awareness	Infertility
Increased digestion	Stroke

Figure 14: The fight-or-flight response is a hard-wired response to stress. The functions listed on the left side of this diagram labeled "Acute stress/rapid/transient" depict instantaneous responses that the cells undergo to fight or flee from a predator or significant threat. The functions listed on the right side labeled "Long-term stress/chronic" depict the conditions that result if the body perceives the threat to be long term. This happens in response to emotional and physical stress, chemicals, toxins, synthetic medications, etc. The cells are hard-wired for this response and cannot judge that a stress is not immediately life-threatening. It's all chemistry at this level. Chronic stress activates the conversion of cholesterol into cortisol and prevents the formation of DHEA, testosterone, and estrogen, which causes body dysfunction and hormone imbalances, which lead to many of the diseases depicted on the right side of this diagram.

Why Stress Responses Never Stop

Because survival is the most important function in the body, the fight-or-flight mechanism will not be turned off until the cells are assured that the threat is gone. Today, threats are much different than they were 200,000 years ago. On top of the food chain, threats look like this: lack of sleep, pesticides, food coloring, toxins, processed foods, job stress, excessive work, artificial light, anxiety, chronic illness, raising children in isolation, financial stress, sitting in traffic every morning, and racing against the clock to be on time.

The body perceives today's modern threats as if a predator were chasing it. So being late for work, financial stress, relationship stress, toxins and other dangerous chemicals are perceived on a cellular level as a predator. The chemical reactions that occur in response to being late for work or stuck in traffic are just the same as being chased by a lion on the cellular level even though we process the information using our brain and eyes and conclude there's no real predator. This mechanism is linked to the fear-based thinking I discussed in chapter one. It's ego-driven for the sake of survival on a harsh planet.

Looking at threats close to the top of the food chain, it's a sure bet that several of them are present daily so this mechanism is never shut off for most people. The demand for resources to handle this stress is ever-increasing while the supply is dwindling. (See figure 15).

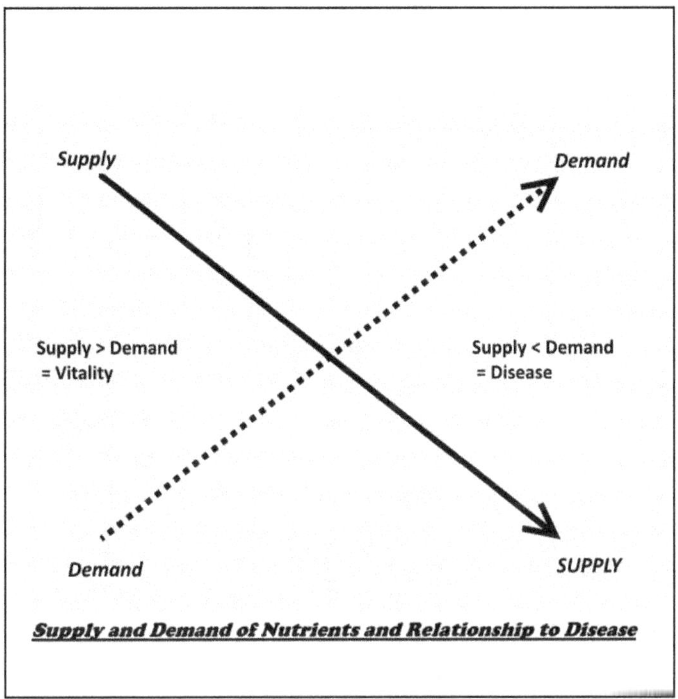

Figure 15: When supply outpaces demand, there are plenty of nutrients and hormones for our cells, and we have great health and vitality. As chronic stress continues, demand for nutrients skyrockets while supply dwindles. As demand outpaces supply, we begin to experience symptoms such as fatigue, weight gain, and brain fog, which can then become diseases such as cancer, heart disease, Alzheimer's dementia, or even autism if it happens early enough in life.

While we have eyes and a brain to perceive and filter things to know that we're not under direct threat, our cells don't have those tools and therefore have an entirely different perception.

Chronic Stress Syndrome

As the body compensates long-term, it begins to reshuffle its resources. This is a self-correcting survival mechanism. As the body scrambles to find a stable point, it sets itself in a dysfunctional place to maintain the peace, compensating and skimping on certain body functions to preserve more important ones.

The survival mechanism of the body requires that it send signals as it shifts things around. These become chronic symptoms, such as fatigue, weight gain, sleep disturbance, low sex drive, poor memory, brain fog, and aches and pains. As we begin to experience these symptoms consistently, we normalize them with our brains so that we can deal with them and keep moving forward. There's no reserve supply available to restore function so body function trickles in a downward spiral just waiting to fall apart.

Given the importance of the adrenal system and its link to many chronic diseases such as cancer and heart attacks, it's critical to have this system properly assessed and treated. Once an adrenal condition is confirmed with TCM as what is called kidney deficiency, specific herbal therapies and nutrition recommendations can be made to help support this system. Cellular-based testing with saliva can confirm the stage of dysfunction, and targeted treatment with nutritional supplements and lifestyle modifications can be implemented.

The adrenal system is slow to recover because it never gets a break. It's equivalent to you breaking your leg but having to walk on it without crutches or braces; it would never properly heal. The adrenal system cannot properly heal without a conscious commitment because stress is unrelenting so it's critical to support this system naturally and specifically gear treatment to each individual's needs. Looking at sources of stress and how to better handle them is critical in healing this system.

Liver Abuse

The body creates waste during its regular body function. This waste is sent to the liver through the venous blood stream. Under normal circumstances, the liver has all the ingredients it needs to neutralize and detoxify all the items that enter the body or are made in the body from everyday living. The liver's job essentially is to change the shape of the things that come to it for elimination through the urine and stools. Once the shape is changed to a form that can leave the body, the liver's job is done as it sends this altered waste to the kidneys and gastrointestinal system to remove them from the body. (See figure 16)

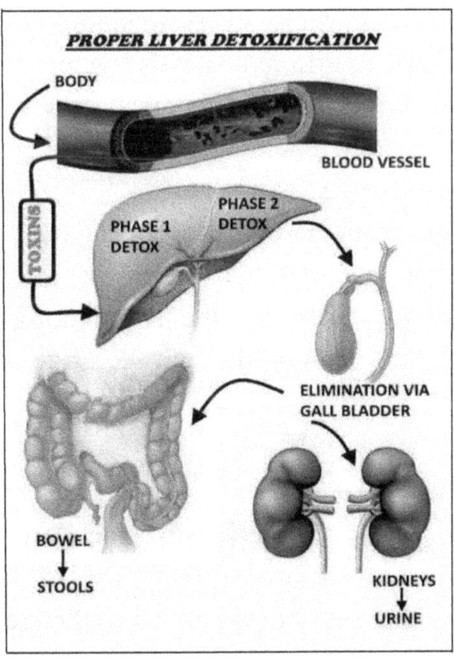

Figure 16: Normal detoxification and elimination of toxins from the body through the bowels and kidneys. If the body is missing key nutrients or if there is an excess of toxins in the body, these dangerous toxins don't leave through the bowels and kidneys and end up back in the body's cells wreaking havoc and causing disease.

Given the environmental changes of the last century, the amount of junk going to the liver has increased substantially, and the form of these toxins is more foreign to the body because they're synthetic or artificial in the vast majority of cases. The liver has to come up with new and creative ways to do its job today and can compensate to a point, but it has its limits.

Today, we're seeing that the liver is running short on what it needs to keep doing this job 24/7 with the new stressors and toxic sludge it has to clean up. The result is that the items are not properly shaped or configured to leave the body and keep recirculating in an altered form because the kidney can't recognize them. This is a form of toxicity. And guess what? Your liver bloodwork will look normal during all this chaos. Now these items are recirculating in altered form and reenter the cells, giving different signals to the cells than they should because they now have a different chemical structure than before. This results in abnormal body function. Over time things start going wrong in the body and lead to diseases.

This is why synthetic hormones, or even your own hormones, can lead to cancer. In the case of your own hormones, it's not the hormones that directly cause the cancer; it's the liver not processing or detoxing them correctly for elimination through the urine or stool that causes problems.

What Synthetic Medications Do to the Liver

Synthetic medications or drugs pose a challenge to the liver. While they may be necessary to save lives, when overutilized, they come at the cost of body function. Most synthetic drugs are of different configurations than natural medicinals found in nature. In order for a drug to be branded, it has to be structurally different than the natural compound. This is how the pharmaceutical industry creates brand drugs. This poses a challenge to the body and the liver in particular, which is in charge of eliminating these compounds from the body.

Our bodies evolved in the environment over thousands of years. Its mechanisms are structured to function according to nature. Although the body can compensate for things that are unnatural, it can't do this long-term without some difficulty. This is why synthetic medications are best used short-term or not at all, if possible.

Once we start using them long-term, the body begins to decompensate. As the liver processes these synthetic drugs, it has to go to more extremes to figure out how to transform the compounds into configurations that can be eliminated from the body. This leads to inflammation and toxicity over time. This can also be recognized as medication side-effects. Many people assume that toxins automatically leave the body without effort, but it's the liver that works to assure this and when it's overworked for too long, it just keep up the pace and toxins accumulate and cause significant problems.

How Liver Dysfunction Leads To Disease

As the liver gets overwhelmed, more and more compounds get missed and don't get changed into the proper configurations or forms to leave the body. Other organs in the body then have to deal with these altered compounds day in and day out. The cells get more of their share of toxins to deal with while trying to maintain body function. The liver runs out of resources when it is overworked and under-supplied.

One critical function of the liver is hormone detoxification or metabolization. This assures proper elimination of hormones through the kidneys and the bowels once they're used. When this doesn't happen, abnormal-looking hormones recirculate in the body. They then return to the cells, giving wrong signals, which result in the wrong work being done by the cell. Over time, this becomes disease. Hormone function is very precise as I'll explain in Chapter 15.

Why Liver *Bloodwork* Is Usually Normal When Liver *Function* Is Not

The explanation lies in the body's survival mechanisms. The body knows that it must maintain normal blood flow for survival. It also knows that it can take from less important cells to maintain this normal blood flow. The result is normal bloodwork and *abnormal* cells.

TCM Explanation of the Liver

Liver is an energy field in TCM. It has many functions not recognized in conventional allopathic medicine. In TCM, liver stores and regulates blood circulation according to physical activity. When we're active, liver releases more blood into circulation to support that activity. When we're at rest, liver stores more blood. Under chronic stress, liver is activated in TCM, resulting in liver stagnation or congestion. This is somewhat equivalent to toxicity in allopathic medicine and can lead to inflammation. Liver in traditional Chinese medicine can also transform or generate heat, which is more or less equivalent to overacidity in allopathic medicine.

Processes that consume blood such as menstruation, pregnancy, breast feeding, and stress, can lead to liver blood deficiency, which then leads to blood deficiency symptoms, such as fatigue, abnormal menstrual cycles, depression, or dizziness. These symptoms are also very similar to liver stagnation or toxicity symptoms, so *similar symptoms can be the result of opposite causes*. Fatigue, for example, can be caused by deficiency of nutrients or by an excess of toxins. So, it's essentially impossible to treat based on symptoms alone and a comprehensive evaluation is needed to distinguish which root causes are at work so that the correct treatment plan is determined.

To Detox Or Not To Detox?

Since symptoms of liver toxicity and deficiency are noticeably similar, it's difficult to know if the treatment should consist of detoxification or tonification through the replenishment of nutrients. These are drastically different principles in TCM.

Detoxification or cleansing is quite draining, and if the patient is deficient or depleted of nutrients, the deficiencies will be worsened by this draining process unless there's proper support. For example, if someone has fatigue due to numerous nutrient deficits that are causing liver toxicity, cleansing or detoxing the liver will result in yet more nutrient deficits, make the patient more tired, and lead to more toxic accumulation over time. This sets up a vicious circle of toxicity with worsening nutrient deficits which will lead to worsening fatigue over time even if the patient feels better initially after temporarily ridding herself of the toxic load. Immediately following the cleanse, you may feel better, but the symptoms will soon recur as the toxins build up again. Why? Because the cause of the toxin build-up is actually the nutrients missing from the liver that make it harder and harder for it to do its job. Cleansing or detoxing without support would simply result in toxicity building up all over again and at the same time draining the valuable nutrients that are in short supply. This approach would not be considered a good solution and many of my patients fall into this trap before coming to see me. I'll call this next client Lisa to conceal her identity. Lisa came to me feeling exhausted all the time. She would read up on the internet and buy liver cleanses that promised that she'd feel better. She would use them faithfully and feel better for a few days and then crash again. She assumed it was because she didn't do enough liver cleanse, so she bought more and did several in a row, which left her feeling even more exhausted than before. She had stopped exercising, wasn't going out with friends as often, had difficulty concentrating at work, and felt dizzy when she stood up too quickly. Lisa had already been to her primary care physician who had no answers for her after doing an extensive panel of blood work. I evaluated Lisa using TCM and diagnosed her with liver qi stagnation against a background of liver blood deficiency. To further evaluate her I asked her to complete a micronutrient panel which revealed 11 cellular nutrient deficits. Lisa consulted with our registered dietician to balance her diet to include the nutrients she was missing. I also prescribed a supplement regimen to more rapidly increase these levels. Lisa had been under significant work stress and we discussed lifestyle modifications to reduce her stress. Lisa felt much better by her one-month follow-up and was back to the gym exercising and participating more fully in her life. Lisa is the perfect example of how the better solution in the face of toxin buildup from nutrient deficits is to correct the nutrient deficits so the liver can do its work.

The key is to know if the liver needs nourishment or if it needs draining/detoxification. TCM answers this question easily.

Determining the Proper Way To Restore Liver Function

Restoring liver health is one of the keys to wellness in the 21st century. Although we can't control all the toxins in our environment from day to day, we can control how our liver responds and recovers to keep our bodies clean.

If the liver is deficient, we should nourish it with proper nutrients. Certain Chinese herbal remedies can be used once the specific patterns of liver blood deficiency are determined. An example of a liver nourishing herb is *dang gui* (*radix angelicae sinensis*). The chief Chinese herbal formula for liver blood deficiency is *si wu tang*, and many other formulas are based on this principle formula. Using cellular-based testing, nutrient deficiencies can be treated with targeted nutrients. Examples are CoQ10, lipoic acid, and B vitamins. If the liver is stagnant or toxic, we should cleanse it with acupuncture, herbs, or detoxification/cleansing systems appropriate for the toxins involved. This helps restore balance and equips the liver to be ready for what comes next. Another client I'll call Donna came to see me for fatigue. She was gaining weight, tired especially in the mornings, and often fell asleep at her desk and had to stand up and move around frequently to stay awake. I evaluated Donna using TCM and diagnosed liver qi stagnation. Donna also had a genetic variation called MTHFR that made liver detoxification more difficult in general. I also tested Donna for heavy metals to assure they weren't a cause of her liver congestion and toxicity. Thankfully, there was no heavy metal toxicity in her case. I prescribed a Chinese herbal formula called Chai Hu Shu Gan Tang did several weekly acupuncture sessions. Donna felt much better in a month. I suggested to her that she do mild liver cleanses once or twice a year to keep the liver functioning more optimally. I also advised her to avoid processed folic acid sources such as found in cereals given her MTHFR gene variant.

Donna and Lisa both had fatigue, but have two completely different root causes or patterns of disharmony, and therefore, their treatments are drastically different. In TCM, a very balanced detoxification can be achieved in a personalized fashion once the pattern of disharmony is determined. This is a very safe way to remove toxins from the body while properly supporting the body's energy. In functional medicine, there are various detoxification or cleansing methods. These are not as customized or personal as TCM methods and can be over-utilized and may cause more harm than good as we saw in Lisa's case before she came to see me. It's critical to have guidance when you believe you have toxins so that you properly regain balance and harmony.

Thyroid Controversies

The thyroid is a key metabolic organ located in your neck. It makes four different hormones to help regulate every aspect of your body's function from heartbeat, breathing, thinking, digestion, reproduction, movement, sleep, and more. It's pretty important. People with an underactive thyroid often feel tired, gain weight, have low sex drive, erectile dysfunction, infertility, constipation, dry skin, and hair loss. These symptoms overlap those of adrenal fatigue that we discussed earlier. People with thyroid disease are also at increased risk for heart disease and cancer.

Two main thyroid hormones are T4 and T3. T4 is known as tetraiodothyronine, and T3 is known as triiodothyronine. T4 is a stored, inactive form of thyroid hormone that must be converted *inside your cells* to its active form called T3. T4 travels in the bloodstream after being made in the thyroid gland and is converted to T3 on an as-needed basis inside your cells to produce thyroid function. Some of this T3 is released into the bloodstream to be taken where it's needed. This can be measured in the bloodstream.

The Forgotten Hormone

When thyroid testing is performed in allopathic medicine, standard of care is to check TSH and free T4 levels with blood work. The word "free" here means that it's a hormone that is not bound in the bloodstream but is available to go into the cells.

TSH is a hormone made in the brain in response to low circulating levels of T4, which is the inactive thyroid hormone. The brain makes more TSH in order to trigger the thyroid gland to make more T4 when blood levels decline. TSH measurement is an indirect testing method that misses a key property: whether or not you have enough *active* T3 hormone *in your cells* where it works in the first place. Another less obvious issue is that your brain actually depends on the thyroid to function properly itself so if the thyroid isn't working right, the brain may not realize it.

Free T4 is the amount of *stored* hormone floating in the bloodstream. This measurement is also indirect because it misses that same key property: whether or not you have enough active thyroid hormone, free T3, in your cells.

Free T3 is the most important thyroid hormone for thyroid function, and it's not tested in allopathic medicine. This leads to millions of people with symptoms of underactive thyroid being improperly diagnosed or not treated. Often TSH and T4 are normal when tested despite the clear presence of thyroid symptoms. Why is that?

Stress and the Thyroid

Stress is likely the most significant cause of what's called "low T3 syndrome." Low T3 syndrome occurs when your free T3 levels are too low, but free T4 and TSH are normal. *Cortisol, the main stress hormone, directly prevents the conversion of T4 to T3.* (See Figure 17.)

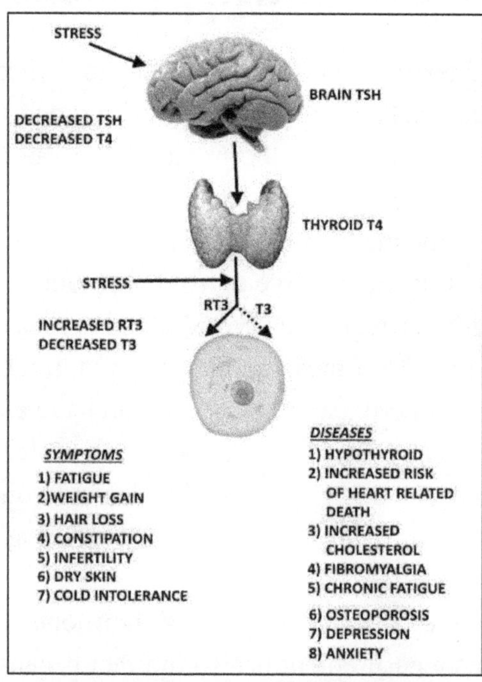

Figure 17: Chronic stress causes decreased TSH (thyroid stimulating hormone). This hormone is responsible for triggering the formation of T4. Decreased TSH then results in decreased T4. Stress also causes T4 to be converted to reverse T3, which is an inactive form of thyroid hormone, rather than T3, which is the active form of thyroid hormone used in the cells. The symptoms of stress-induced low thyroid function are depicted on the left of this diagram, and the diseases that this causes are depicted on the right side of this diagram.

This means that your thyroid is suppressed and doesn't function correctly under stress. Your brain then perceives that all is well because the T4 level is normal so it stops triggering the thyroid to make more T4. **What your brain doesn't know is that cortisol is preventing that T4 from becoming activated into T3**! This makes sense when we look at evolution. In times of fight-or-flight, the adrenal system takes over to raise blood pressure, blood sugar, and heart rate. The thyroid isn't needed for these functions under stress so it's suppressed on purpose and many important functions that are controlled by the thyroid get "turned off" as the body thinks it's tending to much more important problems.

Remember, your cells can't differentiate types of stress; they only know everything is life-threatening because they can't read the memo from your brain that says it's not life-threatening. It's just traffic or your annoying boss, but your cells will never know that. As you begin to have symptoms of underactive thyroid over time, your bloodwork looks normal as usual. It's hard to reduce stress in today's modern times. We live in an era of chronic stressors so it's difficult for the thyroid to pick up its function without significant long-term help to mitigate stress. Treatment may include thyroid hormone replacement of both T4 *and T3*.

Medications that contain both T3 and T4 are available and have been on the market for decades but aren't used by allopathic physicians. Underactive thyroid is classically treated by allopathic medical doctors with levothyroxine (Synthroid®) which is T4 only. The problem with this approach is if you have a suppressed thyroid due to chronic stress, your T4 levels will be normal because you're taking the medication, but your free T3 levels, which aren't measured by conventional allopathic testing, may be lower than normal or low-normal. Your bloodwork will look great, but you won't feel good at all. Your symptoms of underactive thyroid will persist, as will your risk of diseases that come from this metabolic deterioration. Even when properly tested, sometimes the free T3 level is technically normal, but well below average. Integrative and functional medical doctors will treat this with natural thyroid replacement if symptoms are present. In today's stressful environment, having thyroid function that's well below average can lead to unnecessary symptoms and even increase the risk of disease.

Thyroid Toxic Medications

Stress isn't the only factor that causes a suppressed thyroid. Certain medications also prevent conversion of T4 to T3. Some medications that prevent proper thyroid conversion include glucocorticoids, the cardiac medications amiodarone and beta blockers, and synthetic progestins. The list of medications, environmental and natural agents that alter thyroid function is too long to list here. For a detailed discussion, I invite you to read Dr. David Sarnes article, "Effects of the Environment, Chemicals and Drugs on Thyroid Function" in the Journal *Endotext*, last updated in 2016. He is the medical director of the Endocrinology clinics of the University of Chicago.

Iodine and Nutrient Deficiencies

The thyroid relies on many nutrients to produce thyroid hormones. Deficiencies of iodine, lipoic acid, and certain minerals will make it difficult for the body to produce its thyroid hormones and will lead to low thyroid production and symptoms.

Correcting these deficiencies will go a long way to help the body make its own thyroid hormones, but it's important to remember that stress will always place a limit on the production of active thyroid hormone. Despite all that support, your thyroid still may not function normally because cortisol will prevent T3 from being made from T4. It's important to consider thyroid hormone replacement with T4 *and* T3 under these circumstances, or normal thyroid function just won't happen. It's also critical to look at the stressors in your life and begin to mitigate their impact with consistent stress-reduction techniques as discussed in this book.

Also keep in mind that high levels of certain nutrients can also impact thyroid function. Overconsumption of iodine leading to high levels is also detrimental to thyroid function. Remember that balance is the key. In the next chapter, I'll discuss some important misconceptions about vitamins and nutrients you should know.

CHAPTER FOURTEEN

VITAMIN CONTROVERSIES DEMYSTIFIED

Nutritional supplements are more important than ever in today's society, and yet they're so misunderstood. Even worse, they're falsely blamed for causing many medical conditions, including cancer. The beneficial effects of vitamins, minerals, and antioxidants are clearly known based on physiology, which is the study of body function. We know how the body works and how it depends on vitamins, minerals, and antioxidants for its function. There's no confusion here – these facts are taught in medical school using well-researched physiology textbooks. We know the physiological functions of vitamins and minerals based on decades of physiology studies. The National Library of Medicine and the National Institutes of Health confirm the functions of vitamins, minerals, and antioxidants for proper body function.

Nutritional supplements are needed for many reasons. Due to stress and toxins in our environment and soil, today's demands are much higher than past generations. Toxins generated within the body by stress are also an important reason why nutritional supplements are necessary today. We're up and about longer, we sleep less, and this causes the body to use more fuel and nutrients. If you drive your car more, you have to put more gas in it and do more maintenance with oil and tire changes, or it'll just break down. The body is no different.

Our food supply is poor based on numerous studies that show significant drops in nutrients, especially minerals, over the past few decades. This makes it critical for us to replace these nutrients in the form of nutritional supplements when needed.

Why Vitamin Studies Don't Reveal the Truth

Studies on vitamins are mixed at best. Some studies say don't waste your money, and others say vitamins are invaluable. Some even suggest that vitamins and antioxidants cause cancer! Why are there such discrepancies?

A critical point to make here is that many over-the-counter multivitamins contain *synthetic* or artificial ingredients, and **many medical studies use these synthetic vitamins.** When we use synthetic vitamins to replenish deficient vitamins in the body, the normal physiological functions they generally provide don't occur as expected.

The synthetic or artificial version is chemically and structurally different than natural vitamins found in food. It should be no surprise that synthetic vitamins are toxic. The SELECT studies of 2008 and 2011 published by the *Journal of the American Medical Association,* revealed that *synthetic* vitamin E, dl-alpha tocopheryl acetate, caused an increased risk of prostate cancer. It's important to note that natural vitamin E is "alpha-tocopherol," *NOT* "dl-alpha tocopheryl acetate." Natural vitamin E is made from soybean oil and wheat germ oil and can be found naturally in such foods as avocados. Synthetic or artificial vitamin E is made from PETROLEUM. Yes, synthetic vitamin E is not food, but the stuff you put in your car! (See Figure 18). Unfortunately, the public wasn't told that the vitamin E used in the SELECT study was artificial or synthetic. In fact, they made no differentiation at all leading the public to believe that vitamin E causes cancer when it doesn't. You would only know this important information if you looked at the study directly and looked at the chemical name of the studied nutrient to see that it, in fact, is "dl-alpha tocopheryl acetate" and not natural vitamin E.

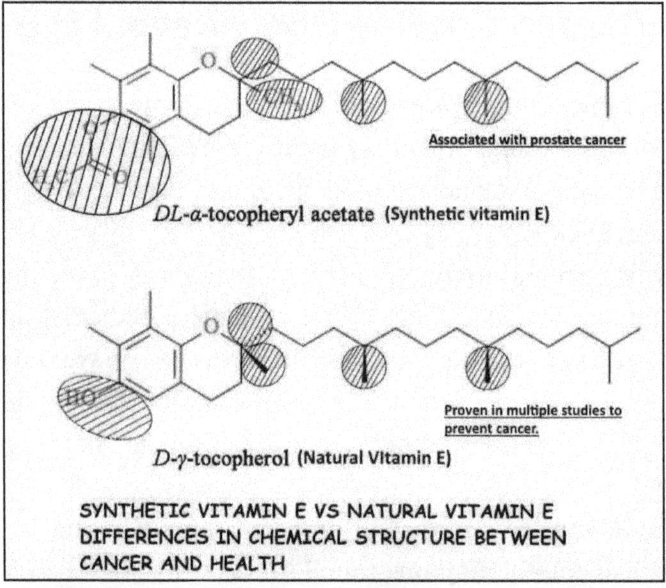

Figure 18: The shaded areas in these illustrations depict the locations on the synthetic and natural vitamin E that differ. There are several locations that are different and this accounts for the differences in their actual functions. Synthetic vitamin E causes cancer and inflammation, whereas natural vitamin E prevents cancer and reduces inflammation.

Thankfully, studies have been done comparing the natural versus synthetic forms of vitamin E. In March 2010, *Archives of Biochemistry and Biophysics* specifically studied the effects of natural and synthetic forms of vitamin E and clearly showed the following: "The data obtained indicates significant qualitative and quantitative differences between the two vitamin forms in regulating gene expression in response to T-cell stimulation. Marker genes have been found whose expression can be considered significant in establishing the level of, and response to vitamin E for both natural and synthetic vitamin E supplementation; unique markers for synthetic vitamin E supplementation and unique markers for natural vitamin E supplementation have been identified."

What this means is that synthetic vitamin E causes your genes or DNA to behave differently than natural vitamin E. This leads to differences in how your immune system cells called T-lymphocytes, which are responsible for fighting cancer, behave! It stands to reason that *synthetic* vitamin E *should not* be used at all! Other studies have been done that link synthetic vitamin E to the following:

- Hemorrhagic stroke
- Increased risk of pneumonia in smokers
- Increased mortality in pancreatic cancer
- Certain radiation-induced skin cancer
- Toxic effect on erythrocytes (red blood cells that carry oxygen)
- Possible contribution to DNA damage in the liver

The good news is that there are natural vitamins available over the counter that are far more useful for the proper function of the immune system and other systems in the body responsible for body function. These allow the body to perform its natural function of defending itself against harmful invaders, such as cancer cells and microbes. The bad news is that there is no requirement for supplement manufacturers to disclose that their vitamins are artificial and you wouldn't know just by reading the label. This is where the guidance of a board-certified integrative medical doctor is critical because we have the ability to distinguish the ingredients of the supplement manufacturers that we recommend to our clients. Alternatively, you can call the manufacturer of a nutrient you intend to use and ask for their documentation of ingredients in what's called a certificate of analysis, but there's still no requirement for them to document that the ingredients are synthetic or artificial on these certificates.

A second critical fact to know is that studies on vitamins usually just focus on one vitamin for its effects. Then that vitamin is judged to be either useless or toxic. There's a very important reason for this: vitamins don't work alone. The body is very complex, and a variety of different vitamins and minerals, antioxidants, and other nutrients are critical for proper body function. If someone is low on one vitamin, chances are they're low on several, and if these aren't corrected, body function won't improve.

Worse yet, if we only prescribe one vitamin, we may imbalance the body further by aggravating the other nutrient deficiencies that are not being addressed and cause more toxicity, such as seen in multiple studies. One important reason the synthetic version of vitamin E causes toxicity is because it reduces or imbalances another natural form of vitamin E needed in the body called gamma tocopherol. This reduction in gamma tocopherol is what is believed to cause the main toxicity seen with synthetic vitamin E.

The *Equine Veterinarian Journal* published a study in 2006 showing that synthetic vitamin E reduces levels of beta carotene, a form of vitamin A which is a critical antioxidant, and worsens oxidative stress in horses after exercise making it more difficult for them to recover.

Synthetic vitamin E was studied and shown to increase the risk of prostate cancer. We know that natural vitamin E doesn't cause prostate cancer. A critical point to make here is that the study fails to indicate that the vitamin E studied was synthetic, and therefore, it blames natural vitamin E for prostate cancer when natural vitamin E helps prevent prostate cancer. The increased risk of cancer is more a function of the synthetic nature of vitamins and the imbalance that was already present in the body. It's likely that many other nutrients were deficient in these patients increasing their risk of cancer. Using only one vitamin drives the body out of balance and creates potential for more problems. Using synthetic vitamins is even more dangerous and potentiates the effects.

A third issue with studies on vitamins is that in some studies a generic multivitamin was prescribed without testing the subject for deficiency prior to prescribing it. The CDC reports that less than 10% of the U.S. population have nutrient deficits, but we have to ask ourselves how they measured this data to come to this conclusion. They use blood levels of nutrients which we're finding out are not accurate assessments of nutrient status for the reasons we discussed in chapter nine. Additionally, blood levels reflect immediate consumption of nutrients and don't give us a steady state or average level. This is very deceiving because blood levels can vary significantly from blood draw to blood draw depending on what you ate or what vitamins you may have taken before having your blood drawn. Looking inside of cells, however, gives us a much more stable and reliable level of nutrients. Medical studies don't measure inside cells so they don't have the correct starting point to conduct their studies.

The World Health Organization published a paper in 2012 comparing blood levels of folic acid to cellular levels and determined that cellular levels were more accurate. The CDC uses blood levels and tells us it's fairly rare for Americans to have nutrient deficits, and this is misleading. As a board-certified integrative medical doctor, I use cellular-based testing to determine nutrient needs and it's exceedingly rare that my clients DON'T have at least 2 or more nutrient deficits. We often see B12 blood levels, for example, being normal while cellular levels are low. It stands to reason that if you're deficient in vitamins other than the ones being given, you won't see any benefit. Additionally, if you're not deficient in the vitamins being given, you won't see the benefits. If you overfill your gas tank and the gas falls on the ground, you won't get any further in your car than if you filled it to the tank's capacity. Further, no multivitamin contains all known vitamins, minerals and antioxidants, so knowing which deficiencies you have is critical to determine which multivitamin or combinations will best correct your deficits. This data is also critical to know when conducting medical studies so that we get accurate data from which to guide our medical protocols.

The fourth reason studies on supplements are misleading is that today's over-the-counter multiple vitamins contain inflammatory fillers that make it very difficult for the vitamin to be absorbed through the intestines so they don't end up in the cells where they belong and are needed. Some multiple vitamins contain dairy, soy, food coloring, and preservatives, and this prevents proper absorption into the body and can also cause inflammation.

One popular over-the-counter multivitamin lists the following "inactive" ingredients on its label: Ascorbyl palmitate, cellulose, citric acid, crospovidone, gelatine (bovine and poultry), glucose, lactose, magnesium stearate, maltodextrin, orange dye, silicon dioxide, sodium ascorbate, sodium benzoate, sodium citrate, sorbic acid, soybean oil, starch, stearic acid, sucrose, and syloid. As a comparison, one of the supplements I recommend to patients contains the following "inactive" ingredients: Natural Vegetable Capsules, Stearic Acid, and Magnesium Stearate. You'll note that in the second supplement, only three additional ingredients are included as opposed to the 20 found in the popular over-the-counter vitamin.

A fifth reason for the current vitamin controversy is that over-the-counter multiple vitamins are often formulated based on outdated government data which is decades old. This is called the Recommended Daily Allowance (RDA). It no longer reflects today's needs. For example, the recommended daily allowance for vitamin D is only 400 units. We know based on new studies that 4,000 units or more are needed to maintain proper levels of vitamin D today. That's 10X the RDA. Certain over-the-counter multivitamins contain only 200 units of vitamin D which would do nothing to prevent deficiencies.

A sixth reason is that many over-the-counter multiple vitamins don't contain what the label says they contain. Given that it's an unregulated industry, many vitamin producers cut corners and don't really give the consumer what's on the label. A review done in 2011 revealed that one-third of 38 nutritional supplements tested didn't contain what was indicated on the label. One way to assure you are getting what's on the label is to ask for a certificate of analysis which is done by an independent lab. This won't guarantee that the ingredients are natural, but it will help you know that the dosing on the bottle is accurate.

Perhaps the most important reason that vitamin studies don't reveal the truth is that many over-the-counter multiple vitamins contain synthetic vitamins, and as previously stated, there's no government requirement to reveal this critical fact. If you look at the label, it simply reads "vitamin E," and you're left to wonder if it's natural or synthetic. You'd have to call the manufacturer and ask for the chemical structure, then compare it to the natural vitamin's chemical structure to assure they are EXACTLY the same.

Many people suffer from nutrient deficiency symptoms and aren't treated, or they're incompletely treated because the testing isn't available in allopathic medicine. Blood work is limited to being able to test for a few nutrient levels and can't reveal cellular levels. Worse yet, vitamins are demonized and blamed for many medical conditions, especially cancer. We can check a few vitamins, such as B12, vitamin D, and folic acid, but no comprehensive cellular panel is available in allopathic medicine to truly determine the needs of each individual. We would have to turn to the field of integrative medicine to obtain this critical cellular testing.

Pesticides and Rapid Farming Impact on Food Quality

Pesticides put in foods since the 1950s are being shown in studies to cause not only toxins to accumulate in our food but also deficiencies in soil quality. Soil is a living organism and is an ecosystem – it contains delicately balanced microorganisms such as bacteria and fungus just like our own gastrointestinal systems. Rapid farming depletes nutrients, especially minerals, in soil because the soil is farmed too quickly, and there's no time for the nutrients in the soil to be replenished. This causes the foods grown in that soil to have deficiencies of nutrients, and when you eat them, you don't get the benefit that you should. We also lose the microorganisms that balance and nourish the soil, which spells disaster for our food supply and environment.

Pesticides also cause nutrient deficiencies in the liver and gastrointestinal tract, the principal detoxification organs for the body. The liver has to work hard when exposed to the chemicals found in artificial pesticides, and this adds up over time, as we discussed before. The liver can become toxic and low in key nutrients it uses to function.

If the liver isn't replenished with the nutrients that it needs, you become toxic and depleted at the same time. This leads to diseases over time. Pesticides are now being recognized as human carcinogens or cancer-causers. The gastrointestinal tract serves an even larger role of detoxification, and pesticides destroy the delicate balance of bacteria needed in the gut for proper function, as we discussed in chapter eleven.

Determining your nutrient requirements is tricky and should be done under the guidance of an integrative physician well versed in TCM and cellular-based testing to drill down into your cells to know your nutrient needs. You should also be guided in picking the right supplements that contain natural nutrients from a trusted source.

I said earlier that vitamins don't work alone. Hormones use nutrients to control body functions. I'll discuss this in the next chapter.

CHAPTER FIFTEEN

HORMONES: FRIEND OR FOE?

The Truth About Hormones

Hormones are the body's blueprints. They tell all 100 trillion cells of your body how to function. Hormones even tell your cells when to make more hormones, so hormones regulate every aspect of body function. There are hundreds of different types of hormones in the human body, and each type is responsible for different functions.

Hormones are made by the body as needed and are used in the body's cells. They are "disposable," and once used in the cell, must be eliminated from the body by the liver and kidneys. Hormones should never be used twice. For example, estradiol is primarily made in the ovaries. It's considered the "female hormone" and is responsible for up to 400 different body functions in both men and women.

Hormones called FSH (follicle stimulating hormone) and LH (luteinizing hormone) are hormones responsible for estrogen production in the cells of the ovaries. Once an estradiol molecule is made in the ovaries and released into the bloodstream, it goes into the cells through estrogen receptors and regulates the cells' functions. Cells have receptors that are like windows that open to allow hormones to enter the cell. The hormone is transported into the nucleus, or command center, of the cell where it's read like a blueprint by the cell's mechanisms.

The hormone has to enter the cell to function. While the hormone's in the bloodstream, it's simply being transported from one place to another and has minimal function. The amount of hormone in the bloodstream does have some effect in hormone regulation and synthesis of new hormones, but the hormones being made don't function until they're brought inside the cells. If the body is short on the ingredients that make hormones due to various reasons, then it won't make sufficient hormones and cells will be deprived if they're not high enough on the food chain.

The cell responds to hormones by turning on various genes and turning off others. Each gene regulates a particular function in the cell. Without hormones, the cell doesn't know which genes to turn on or off and may very well turn on the wrong genes, or fail to turn on critical genes that are needed for body function. Given our growing information about the precision of the genetic code in the body, we're realizing that even the slightest variation of the chemical structure of hormones is critical to body function.

The hormone I mentioned earlier, estradiol, for example, has *400 different functions in the human body* in *both* men and women. Once the cell uses that estrogen, it's released from the receptor and goes to the liver. It enters the liver cells, which then change its appearance using chemical reactions called conjugation and methylation. This is part of the detoxification function of the liver. These reactions are critical for changing estradiol's appearance so that it can be eliminated from the body through the kidneys via urination. That estradiol molecule should never go back into the body once it has entered the liver. When the body needs more estradiol, the ovaries are stimulated to make more. There's a very specific and critical reason for this that I'll explain in a bit. Hormones dictate cellular function. Diseases occur when cells don't function properly. Stress can cause hormone imbalances that lead to cellular and body dysfunction and eventually diseases.

How Stress "Stresses Out" Your Hormones

Cortisol released by the adrenal glands in response to chronic stress, impacts insulin, which is the hormone that regulates blood sugar. Cortisol causes increases in blood sugar. Chronic stress can cause persistent elevations in blood sugar, leading to insulin resistance, which is a precursor to diabetes.

Cortisol impacts the thyroid and suppresses its production of hormones, leading to low thyroid function; this causes fatigue, weight gain, and many other disturbances of body function.

Cortisol also impacts the hormone progesterone because progesterone is used to make cortisol. When there's too much stress, progesterone will become depleted as it's used to make more and more cortisol. High cortisol produced during stress will also block progesterone receptors on your cells leading to the inability of the cell to use progesterone even if it's present in the blood stream. Why? Nature is smart. It knows that if you're being threatened by a predator or other life-threatening situation, you shouldn't reproduce or your vulnerable offspring will be in danger. Again, nature didn't intend for the fight-or-flight reactions to be chronic as they are today. Chronic stress is a man-made phenomenon. A lack of progesterone is dangerous in the long run as progesterone balances estrogen. Estrogen dominance, which occurs when progesterone is too low for good balance, causes excessive cellular growth, which can increase the risk of cancer.

Stress also causes liver nutrient deficiencies when it becomes too chronic. This leads to hormone changes as well. For example, vitamin B6 (pyridoxine) deficiency can cause excess estrogen, whereas vitamin B2 (riboflavin) reduces estrogen levels. If these critical vitamins are out of balance, your estrogen will also be out of balance.

Why Our Hormones Go Out of Balance

Chronic stress causes hormone imbalances because stress isn't supposed to be chronic. Stress should be a short-lived physiological response to threats. Today, things are different, and our evolutionary survival mechanisms don't work for our *chronic* stressors. Hormone imbalances are perpetuated by the cells' perceptions that the body is under threat. For example, cortisol is made from progesterone. Progesterone has many different functions in the body, one of which is reproduction. When stress becomes chronic with elevated cortisol levels, progesterone declines as it's siphoned off to make cortisol. This leads to menstrual abnormalities and infertility. Nature has built-in protective mechanisms to assure that we don't reproduce under threatening situations. Progesterone deficiencies have also been shown in studies to cause miscarriages and premature fetal deliveries. Again, the cells have no means of telling the difference between you being angry about sitting in traffic or really being under threat, so any perceived long-term stress can cause significant abnormalities that are not recognized by conventional allopathic medicine, leaving millions of people without answers.

An imbalance of cortisol that results from stress causes a host of other problems that are beyond the scope of this book, but many hormone imbalances result from chronic stress as we've already discussed. Long-term hormone imbalances can lead to diseases. Why is this? Our own hormones can turn against us under chronic stress. As stress becomes chronic, it causes the body to use up more nutrients. The liver becomes overwhelmed in its function as it runs out of nutrients and builds up toxins.

Our liver is principally responsible for breaking down our hormones so that they can be eliminated. Remember that hormones are disposable – after being used, they go to the liver for detoxification and eventual elimination. There's a good reason for this process. If the liver doesn't do its job, the hormones enter the liver and are altered in their appearance but *not in a way that they can be eliminated from the body*. In other words, *the blueprint is changed, and those hormones recirculate in the body instead of being eliminated and they remain in a toxic form*.

As we learned earlier, this isn't a good thing. Blueprints that aren't made by nature can be dangerous. We're learning about this more and more now that we've mapped out our DNA and genes. We're learning just how precise gene function is. Instead of being eliminated from the body, the hormones recirculate in the body and end up in our cells all over again and deliver a different message than they should, and this leads to the wrong genes being turned on and off, leading to diseases long-term. Hormone *imbalances* are essentially the same as taking synthetic hormones: bad news.

Toxin accumulation is another reason our own hormones turn against us. The liver can only do so much. In today's environment, there are hundreds of toxins that weren't present even a hundred years ago: household cleaning products, pesticides, plastics, makeup, and synthetic drugs. These all compete with your hormones for conjugation and methylation reactions in order to be eliminated from the body. In other words, there's a lot of competition for detoxification in the liver these days. If the liver's overloaded, certain substances won't be properly handled by the liver and will spill back into the body. This means that toxins will be recirculating in the body rather than being removed from the body. This also means that hormones will have the same fate, recirculating in the body in toxic form wreaking havoc on body function.

Why Synthetic Hormones Are Toxic

Hormone function and structure are very precise. A glaring example is natural progesterone versus the synthetic version called medroxyprogesterone acetate (MPA). MPA is an artificial hormone contained in a drug called Prempro®, which is used for hormone replacement therapy in the United States. The Women's Health Initiative study released in 2004 revealed an increased risk of breast cancer and stroke in women taking Prempro® for more than 5 years.

Progesterone, which is a natural hormone produced by the body, causes no toxicity in the human body and has not been linked to an increased risk of breast cancer or stroke. After all, nature created it specifically *for* our bodies. It's been shown to *reduce* the risk of breast cancer, and recent studies are beginning to link progesterone deficiency with Alzheimer's dementia. There's no association between natural progesterone and any chronic diseases.

The synthetic hormone, medroxyprogesterone acetate, on the other hand, has been clearly linked to an increased risk of breast cancer and stroke. Why? If you look at the structure of natural progesterone versus medroxyprogesterone acetate, they're not the same (see figure 19).

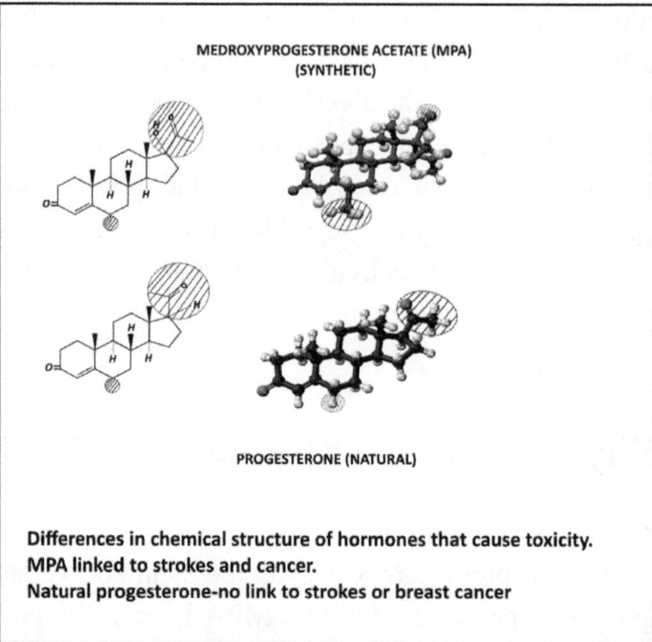

Figure 19: The shaded areas in these illustrations of medroxyprogesterone acetate (MPA) and natural progesterone depict the locations on these molecules that are different. The differences in their chemical structure don't seem like much, but the effects of synthetic progesterone are disastrous, increasing the risk of strokes and breast cancer, as compared to natural progesterone, which is protective and shows no link to strokes or breast cancer.

Medroxyprogesterone acetate is different than human progesterone, and this is critical reason why it's toxic. Nature put in place all that was needed for the human body when it evolved in its environment. The body's DNA was clearly designed to assure proper body function in the environment in which the human body evolved.

When we change the plan that nature puts in place, bad things happen. When we take a drug such as medroxyprogesterone acetate, we're allowing a synthetic hormone with a different blueprint to enter the body and its cells. Once within the cells, medroxyprogesterone acetate will cause the cells to activate or inactivate genes they're not supposed to, and this leads to disease or death over time.

Because the effects are not immediate, it can be difficult to see the link unless studies such as the Women's Health Initiative bring this to light. **The common denominator to many of these dangerous drugs is their artificial or synthetic nature** – studies aren't really needed to surmise this. This is simply the logical conclusion from putting things in the body that don't belong there. At first, as cells do the wrong thing, the body can compensate for this, and we feel fine. As the burden increases over time — day after day, year after year — the body can no longer compensate for incorrect body function, and cancers and strokes can occur as the body finally decompensates under this pressure. *It's important to remember that cells have no eyes or brains and cannot distinguish minor differences in hormones.* They just do what the chemical structure of the hormone dictates they should do. The cells can't tell that there's a fake hormone dictating body function. It's all chemistry at that level, and cells follow instructions exactly as the blueprint dictates. Why? Again, **nature never intended for the body to have to distinguish this because there are no synthetic hormones in nature.**

This is the reason why the Women's Health Initiative Study in 2004 concluded that the danger in the use of medroxyprogesterone acetate occurred after five years of use and not immediately. The body can handle a lot, but eventually breaks if it's pushed past its brink.

When natural progesterone is used instead, the body gets the right blueprint and signals so it can turn the correct genes on or off over time, and proper body function is maintained. That's why progesterone has not been linked with chronic diseases or death.

Synthetic hormones are toxic for a second reason. The liver evolved in the human body to eliminate things found in nature once they enter our blood stream. Studies have shown that Premarin®, which is conjugated equine estrogen derived from horse urine, can *linger in the body for as long as six months after the drug is stopped.* That's alarming, but not surprising. With Premarin® we're literally prescribing the toxic version of estrogen removed from the horse through its urine. That's how we eliminate our toxins! It shouldn't be the way we reintroduce them into our bodies! Further, a hormone should be immediately eliminated from the body once used in our cells. The fact that Premarin® lingers for six months after the cessation of its use tells us clearly that it's burdening the liver.

During the menstrual cycle, hormones are made and immediately eliminated, and fresh hormones are made as needed. This is actually what allows for the menstrual cycle to occur as seen in figure 20. If hormones lingered in the body, they would accumulate, and menses would be interrupted. This is, in fact, the mechanism of action of birth control pills and why they work. These contraceptives are synthetic and have different blueprints than natural hormones, causing them to linger in the body, interrupting menses and providing contraception by rendering the woman infertile. Knowing this, it's no surprise that they, too, have been shown in studies to increase the risk of cancer and stroke after 10 years of use. They're probably safer longer because women who use them are generally younger and healthier than women in menopause and can withstand the toxicity.

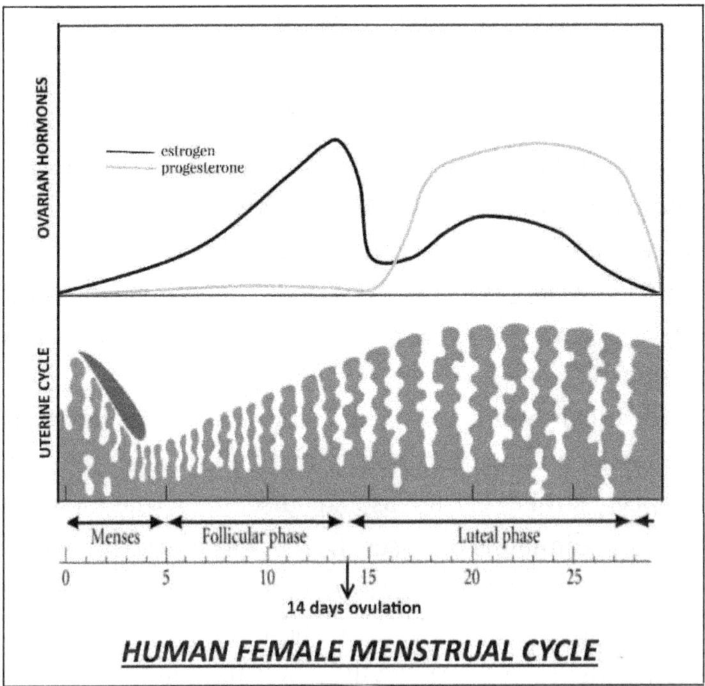

Figure 20: The female menstrual cycle is a complex building-up of the uterine lining followed by either pregnancy or menstruation, depending on whether the ovarian "egg" is fertilized by sperm. The ebb and flow of this cycle is orchestrated by hormones, which are tightly regulated. This illustration shows how the levels of estrogen and progesterone vary throughout the cycle and how this impacts the uterine lining. If these hormones are not properly used and eliminated, the menstrual cycle ceases and infertility results.

When we check our innate hormone levels, they vary and are very cyclic over time. The detoxification of these hormones by the liver followed by elimination by the kidneys is a key function for normal menses and reproduction.

Bio-Identical Hormones

Bio-identical hormone therapy, or BIHT, is a concept developed in Europe and used there extensively for over four decades. BIHT has been studied in Europe for over 20 years with very positive results.

BIHTs have the same blueprint as human hormones. They're plant-based and natural. Most BIHTs are compounded, which means that they are made by certified pharmacists based on a physician's prescription.

Bio-identical hormones have been shown to have significant positive impact on body function. They've been shown to help reduce breast cancer, stroke, cardiovascular disease, Alzheimer's dementia, and certain autoimmune diseases. BIHTs have been shown to improve quality of life, improve longevity, help with weight reduction and maintenance, improve metabolism, and immunity.

Recently the FDA restricted the fillers used in the compounding of bioidentical hormones. When hormones are compounded, they are stabilized in fillers for proper absorption and to preserve them. Previously, bioidentical hormones were stabilized in fillers such as coconut oil or olive oil. The FDA cited shelf-life and stability as a reason to remove these natural fillers from the market forcing some compounding pharmacies to use synthetic fillers. Adding synthetic fillers to natural hormones defeats the purpose and adds toxicity to a treatment that should be healing. *It's critical that you ask your doctor and pharmacist about the fillers being used to assure that one of the few remaining natural fillers is being used in your hormone formulation.*

Safe When Properly Monitored

The use of bio-identical hormones must be monitored for proper safety. When balancing hormones, it's critical to assure that the cells that require these hormones for their function have them in the correct *amounts*. The cell responds to every hormone that enters it so if one estrogen molecule enters, the cell does the work once. If 200 molecules of estrogen enter the cell, the cell does that work 200 times, so it's critical to have the correct *amount* of hormones for proper function. If too much hormone is used, cells can develop resistance to hormones and hide their receptors in an attempt to protect themselves. It's equally important to monitor the proper *removal* of hormones from the body and its cells once they're used.

What Does Proper Hormone Monitoring Mean?

Given that hormone function occurs inside cells, it's critical to *monitor* the levels inside the cells as well. Using bloodwork to monitor hormone replacement therapy can be misleading and potentially dangerous.

A 2012 *New England Journal of Medicine* study concluded that testosterone replacement therapy in older men was associated with a significantly increased risk of cardiovascular events. This study flew in the face of decades of research showing the safety of natural testosterone replacement therapy. The study specifically used testosterone cream, which was applied through the skin. In allopathic medicine, it's falsely assumed that only ten percent of the applied cream will reach the tissues and cells when measured between 12-24 hours after application. Because of this false assumption, the ***FDA-approved dose of testosterone gel is ten times the amount that a healthy young male will produce in a day*****!**

The FDA-approved dose of testosterone gel is 50-100mg per day, whereas a healthy young male produces 5-10mg of testosterone per day. There's a *big difference between what the levels in the bloodstream are when we make our own hormones and when we apply them as a cream.* Studies on cellular levels of testosterone after gel application show levels are 10-20 times higher than blood levels. In other words, the cells are being overdosed with testosterone and are malfunctioning due to this toxic overload. It's not the testosterone that's the problem, it's the amount that's allowed to enter the cells that causes toxicity.

BIHT can take many forms: transdermal creams, oral capsules, pellets, and troches (pronounced trō-kees). Pellets are inserted under the skin, transdermal creams are applied on top of the skin, oral capsules are swallowed, and troches are held between the cheek and gum until dissolved.

How a hormone gets into the body matters. Transdermal *creams* go to the body's *cells* first, then trickle into the bloodstream, and then to the liver. *Oral* hormones go to the *gastrointestinal tract* first, then immediately to the liver, then they go to the body's *cells*.

When taking transdermal creams, it's critical to monitor *cellular* levels since the cells get the bulk of the administered hormones. When you make your *own* hormones, they are released into the *bloodstream* first, then they go to the *cells*, and then to the *liver*. The journey of the hormone varies, and proper monitoring of administered hormones is critical for safe use. This is a significant flaw in studies conducted on hormone creams and gels. It's assumed that all hormones behave the same no matter how they're administered. This is simply not the case.

Cellular-based monitoring helps reduce risks associated with hormone replacement therapy. Cellular-based testing can be done in various ways:

- **Saliva**: Saliva testing has been shown to approximate glandular levels, which reflect cellular levels.
- **Capillary** blood levels: Capillaries are at the level of tissues where groups of cells are located and obtaining samples from capillaries reflects the cellular environment.
- **Urine**: Urine helps determine body *storage* of hormones and is invaluable for determining how the liver is breaking down hormones for *removal* from the body. Elimination of hormones can only be determined using urine. Saliva and capillary sampling don't tell us about proper breakdown and elimination. There are certain breakdown products of hormones that tell us whether or not hormones are being properly eliminated from the body, which urine assessments can disclose.

A Day in the Life of A Hormone

Estradiol hormone is manufactured in the body or taken as hormone replacement therapy. This hormone will travel through the skin and to the cells of the body when taken as a transdermal cream. Estradiol will attach to the cell receptor that is specific for estradiol. For example, estrogen will not bind to a cell receptor that isn't specifically for estradiol. It won't bind to a progesterone receptor, for example.

The receptor will transport estradiol into the cell, and it'll be carried to the cell's nucleus. Once within the nucleus, the cell's mechanism will read the estradiol hormone and perform the functions specifically associated with estradiol. Once used, the estradiol will be transported out of the cell and go to the bloodstream and into the liver. The liver will take in that estradiol and begin the chemical reactions to change estradiol to 2-hydroxyestrone (2-OH-E1), 4-hydroxyestrone (4-OH-E1), and 16-hydroxyestrone byproducts.

The 2-OH E1 and 4-OH E1 byproducts must be further changed through a process called methylation into inert forms called 2- and 4 methoxy-estrogens. These chemical reactions depend on an enzyme called COMT, vitamins B12, folate, and B6. *If there are genetic alterations in COMT or deficiencies of B12, folate, or B6, the byproducts are instead oxidized and become highly toxic*. These toxic oxidized byproducts, called 2-quinone estrogen and 4-quinone estrogen, are highly reactive and *cling to DNA, causing damage*. These toxic byproducts can still be inactivated by an antioxidant called *glutathione* and rendered harmless. However, if glutathione levels are low, these oxidized toxins wreak havoc on DNA, causing gene mutations which predispose to cancer. Glutathione is made in the body in the gastrointestinal tract and liver using various amino acids, vitamins and minerals. Nature actually has many levels of protection in case things go wrong.

Estrogen byproducts will be recognized by the kidney and eliminated from the body through the urine. If urine testing is done, you can have the levels and ratios of these byproducts measured to assure that you are breaking down estradiol properly. Improper metabolization has been linked to breast cancer and other diseases that can kill.

If that estradiol is not completely changed to one of these inert byproducts for elimination, the kidney will not recognize it, and it will keep circulating in the bloodstream and end up in another cell where it will look altered and give the wrong cellular instructions. If you see that the body is getting toxic from this process with proper testing, you can intervene with added nutrients including glutathione to correct the elimination process or stop the hormones as you make these critical corrections.

When Hormones Go Rogue

Hormones can go rogue under certain circumstances:

1. If their levels are too low
2. If their levels are too high
3. If they aren't properly broken down and removed from the body

1. *If their levels are too low:*

If you're not taking or making sufficient amounts of hormones, your body's cells will be left unguided and not function properly. Estrogen deficiency has been linked to Alzheimer's dementia, osteoporosis, cardiovascular diseases, autoimmune diseases, infertility, menstrual abnormalities, hot flashes, fatigue, and memory loss, to name a few. Estrogen is needed for eye function, gut function, muscle mass, bone production, skin maintenance, immune system function, etc. Low levels of estrogen will lead to dysfunction of these systems, even in the absence of disease.

2. *If levels are too high:*

If there's too much of a particular hormone, the cells will be overburdened with work that isn't necessary, and the liver will have to work harder to eliminate these hormones, which can result in recirculating hormones that are toxic.

3.*If they aren't properly broken down and eliminated from the body:*

If the liver is overburdened or depleted, it will not break your hormones down properly, and they will recirculate in toxic form back into the body.

Given this information, it's easy to see how hormones can be misunderstood and misused. If you suspect hormone imbalances may be responsible for your symptoms or conditions, it's critical to obtain an integrative evaluation based on TCM principles and cellular-based testing so you can gain balance and benefit from nature's intended body function.

No discussion on hormones would be complete without a discussion on menopause. In the next chapter, I'll explain menopause from a TCM perspective, which will likely change the way you look at this important time in a woman's life.

CHAPTER SIXTEEN

MENOPAUSE: THE BEGINNING OF THE END?

Menopause: The TCM Explanation

Menopause is a very misunderstood phase of life for women. It's often mistaken as a syndrome because many symptoms pop up during these times that were dormant before. Many women think the terrible symptoms associated with this time of transition are normal, a rite of passage, so to speak. I'm here to tell you that adverse symptoms are anything but normal.

The technical definition of menopause is the cessation of menstruation for over a year. Period…no pun intended! No hot flashes, night sweats, sleep issues, anxiety, depression, weight gain — none of that noise is part of menopause.

TCM helps us better understand menopause and why we're needlessly suffering through it. In TCM, there's a cycle of energy that regulates the menstrual cycle. During the third week of the cycle, the TCM *Liver* meridian is mobilized.

The TCM *Liver* regulates the flow of energy and blood so it mobilizes energy that will, in turn, mobilize the blood downward and outward from the uterus. We recognize this as our menstrual flow.

The TCM *Liver* is also responsible for regulating the amount of blood in circulation. When our activity is increased, the liver releases blood into the circulation to support that activity. When we're at rest, blood returns to the liver to be stored.

When menopause occurs, energy and blood have to make a 180-degree turn. We no longer menstruate so there's no downward and outward flow of blood anymore. Instead, this energy is mobilized upward to nourish the TCM *Heart* meridian. This is why older women are said to have wisdom. If the *Liver* meridian is not harmonized during menopause, symptoms can occur. There can be many reasons why the TCM *Liver* can't regulate the flow of qi during this time. Other organ systems in Chinese medicine are involved, such as the TCM *Heart* and the TCM *Kidney*. In TCM, organs are not physical entities but are *energetic* systems that function throughout the body. For example, in TCM the *Kidney* meridian has multiple functions and maintains the brain, the spinal cord, essence, genetics, bones, teeth, lower body function, and supports many other organ systems as the "root" of the body. The organs we know as the kidneys in conventional medicine are a very small part of the TCM *kidney*. An imbalance in the TCM *Kidney* system can cause an array of symptoms affecting multiple other systems in the body.

Stress-O-Pause: Why Women Feel Like They're Falling Apart During Menopause

There's a critical relationship between stress and menopause. In Chinese medicine, it's well appreciated that the more stress present before menopause, the rockier the transition. This is because stress impacts many organ systems involved in the menopause transition. The body is busy undergoing trillions upon trillions of chemical reactions daily, changing the functions of numerous systems to transition into a completely different phase of life that we know as menopause.

The TCM relationship between stress and menopause is clearly understood. When the liver is not properly functioning — either because it is depleted or stagnant — menopause can be a very difficult experience. In TCM, the *Liver* is known as the stress organ because it can become depleted or stagnant under stressful circumstances. In allopathic medicine we relate stress to the adrenal system. Chronic stress affects the TCM *Kidney*, which is also known as the reserve or root of the body. This explains a lot of symptoms that we experience in menopause — hot flashes, night sweats, sleep disturbances, depression, and anxiety. These symptoms are not a normal part of menopause and should not be experienced during this time.

Even without treatment, these symptoms will eventually subside as the body uses its self-correcting mechanisms to stop these distressing symptoms so we can regain peace. The problem with this is that the trouble is still brewing underneath. The root causes of the symptoms don't get treated. The body simply finds an alternate route to keep the peace. The body can't choose to bypass menopause; it's genetically programmed to happen, so the body will do whatever it has to do to continue the menopause process and also try to stop these distressing symptoms. It does so by short-changing less critical body systems. As the body works hard to compensate, it can eventually *decompensate*, and this is why many diseases are diagnosed during the time of menopause transition. For example, we know that the risk of heart attacks increases in women as they transition through menopause. Women have a natural protection from heart attacks that is distinctly reduced as we transition through menopause. Our risk of heart attack increases to that of men during this time of life.

We can also look at menopause as an opportunity for disease prevention. Many studies are beginning to link midlife stress to breast cancer, coronary artery disease, and Alzheimer's dementia, just to name a few. In other words, the stress you experience in your 40s is responsible for the diseases you get in your 50s and 60s and beyond. Stress isn't going away, but we can definitely do something about its impact on our bodies, minds, and spirits. The Institute of HeartMath® has shown that we can build resiliency against stress. The fields of neurobiology and quantum physics are showing us that we create our realities and can drastically reduce the impact of stress, so there's plenty of evidence that it's doable.

Using the principles that I've discussed in this book, we can begin to see what's really at the root of our symptoms and diseases and begin to shift the paradigm to one that helps mitigate the impact of stress in a more prevention-oriented way. A TCM-based integrative evaluation, combined with cellular-based testing that drills down into your cells for answers, allows you to see your risk and root causes for diseases to correct them. This goes a long way to help reduce symptoms of menopause and most importantly, the diseases that result from these symptoms. In the next chapter, I'll discuss how stress is actually FIXABLE! Knowing this puts YOU in the driver's seat to direct your own wellness.

CHAPTER SEVENTEEN

WHEN THE ULTIMATE ROOT CAUSE IS UNFIXABLE... OR IS IT?

The primary cause of disease and dysfunction within the body today is chronic stress and the changes it causes in the body as its effects rage on for months or years. The human body can only compensate for so much before diseases set in. The problem is stress isn't going anywhere anytime soon. Now what?

The Institute of HeartMath®'s ground-breaking research shows us that stress doesn't have to be our undoing. Harmonization of heart and brain provides resiliency against stress. Using a combined approach of heart-brain harmonization with an integrative holistic approach is a powerful tool and a critical tool for 21st century wellness!

Although we can't make stress go away, *we can determine and control how stress impacts us*. The impact of stress is like a fingerprint. It's unique to each individual. Treating stress and its effects varies for everyone.

Using anxiety medications may be a solution for temporary severe stress relief but not for chronic stress. Using anxiety medications is not only highly addictive, but potentially dangerous. Chronic stress must be treated differently to avoid diseases or deterioration of body function and quality.

Another critical factor is to look to the heart-brain for solutions. The studies done over the past 20-30 years on heart-brain and head-brain harmonization (or coherence) shows us without question that we can build resiliency against stress, mitigate its impact and regain and maintain normal body function and wellness. Engaging a heart-centered lifestyle practice with breathing and self-management programs is a critical path to overcome or circumvent stress as the common denominator of disease.

When the ultimate root cause of disease within the body may seem untreatable because the stressors are still present, providing the body with what it needs to successfully thrive under stress and restore itself while maintaining body function is the secret to wellness in the 21st century environment.

The human body is an elegant, miraculous, and complex machine. When its function is lost or diseases set in, restoring body function is critical to recovery and maintenance of health. The delicate balance that maintains body function must be restored for success. This requires diagnosing and treating root causes of body dysfunction while using heart-brain harmonization to help build resiliency against stress over time.

TCM is one of the most powerful systems of medicine for determining root causes of body dysfunction and disease. Energy-based systems of medicine like TCM should be the starting point for all evaluations of body dysfunction. Once patterns of disharmony are known, we can give powerful personal nutritional and lifestyle guidance to help begin the process of restoring balance and health.

Chinese herbal therapy is a powerful tool to rebalance the body's energy. Heart-centered mindfulness is a powerful tool to rebalance the mind and spirit. The **unseen** functions of the body and its connection to its environment are critical to its restoration. The **visible** pieces that we see and measure are just a small part of body function. The other distinct advantage of TCM and the use of acupuncture and herbal formulas is that we can safely target treatment to a particular system while still supporting the whole body and mind.

With nutrition, supplements, and hormones, as is practiced in functional medicine, the body decides where to send these nutrients *based on demand.* The body's self-correcting mechanisms decide where they're needed most, and the low priority cells have to wait until the other more important cells have what they need. The process can be sped up with the use acupuncture and Chinese herbal therapy so the treatments reach all needed areas as efficiently as possible. With acupuncture and herbs, we can control where the energy and nutrients are sent, which can speed recovery. We have the distinct advantage of drilling deep down into the cellular metabolic mechanisms where energy is produced in order to correct these processes.

There are significant unseen forces at work in the body that TCM can recognize and help balance. Functional medicine is a critical tool that adds cellular and metabolic tests to determine the fine details of body dysfunction for restoration.

If a patient is depleted, they must be replenished with proper nutrients, natural hormones, and rest. Testing is a critical step in determining the specifics required, and it should be cellular-based because that's the only way to know your cells' needs and regain proper body function. Remember the second law of thermodynamics is like gravity. It's always at work! If you don't pump energy back into a system, it deteriorates — plain and simple. Stress uses up a lot of energy and if it's not replenished, you get sick. That's plain and simple, too.

If a patient is toxic or stagnant based on TCM principles, then acupuncture or Chinese herbal formulas can be prescribed. Testing should be geared to finding sources of toxicity, and the patient may be detoxed with acupuncture, herbs, or liver-gut cleanse therapies. Chelation therapy may even be needed if heavy metals are found. Chelation therapy is a safe method of removal of heavy metals such as lead and mercury from the body. Heavy metals are very toxic and have been linked with multiple diseases, especially cancer.

TCM helps us to know which direction to head to restore body function from an energy or metabolic level. TCM helps keep us on track as the body shifts as we recover body function by showing us the energy of the body at work. This mitigates the impact of stress. Stress doesn't just vanish, but we can stay healthy and thrive despite it.

Stress Never Takes A Break So Neither Can We

Keep walking, though there's no place to get to.
Keep walking, though there's no place to get to.
Don't try to see through the distances
That's not for human beings.
Move within but don't move the way fear makes you move.

---Rumi as translated by Coleman Barks

When patients begin to feel better, they mistakenly believe that they can stop using their spiritual practice, heart-brain coherence practice, herbs, and supplements because they feel better. What's critical to know is that they feel better *because* they're providing the body with what it needs despite its stress.

When we stop using the methods that keep us well, the impact of stress begins anew, and our symptoms begin to creep back in. Is it because our treatments aren't effective? No. It's because stress never takes a break. We can't always control the toxins in our atmosphere or in our homes. This keeps stress in our lives no matter what.

Eliminating stress as much as possible is critical, but eliminating it entirely is nearly impossible. Because of this, the days of simply eating well and exercising to maintain the physical body are over. That's no longer enough to maintain wellness in the face of the unprecedented stress we experience today.

Maintaining Normal Function

All bets are off today as our environment has changed drastically, and the human body itself is in a strange place. It has to adapt to this strange place constantly. Proper periodic monitoring and assessment with TCM helps us maintain proper body function once restored. Our needs change over time as we age or encounter different stressors such as changes in environment, medications, or life circumstances. Continued deep listening and going within helps us stay on track to nourish our mind, soul and body. Being vigilant in our monitoring and also consistent in changing our nutrition, exercise, and supplements as needed is equally important. Our dynamic nature requires it to maintain wellness.

The human body is essentially in a foreign environment today, and the **physiological mechanisms of fight-or-flight are completely unchanged**. It would take thousands, if not millions of years to change our genes to change our fight-or-flight responses because we're too complex to change our genetic information quickly. So, we're stuck in our foreign environment UNLESS WE **CHOOSE** TO CHANGE HOW WE **PERCEIVE** STRESS by going within. We can make the best of it thanks to the ancient powerful wisdom of heart-centered living, traditional Chinese medicine, and the leading-edge technology of cellular-based testing as found in integrative/functional medicine. Implementing all this powerful information into our culture is the next step on our journey to wellness.

In the next chapter, I'll propose a radical and bold new way for us to start changing the tide of disease to one of wellness and drastically change our culture from a "sick-care" model to a healthcare model.

CHAPTER EIGHTEEN

THE FUTURE OF HEALTH

Creating A positive Health Experience For Ourselves

Now that we have this wealth of information, what are the first steps to creating good health and feeling good? Feeling good is an experience no one can prove to us until we're there. The fields of integrative and energy-based medicines are often confronted with the argument that there aren't enough studies to support them. The reason that allopathic medical doctors think there are no studies is because the studies are frequently published in journals they don't consistently read. I was surprised to find the most significant medical and scientific studies in *Nature* magazine and *Scientific American*, both peer-reviewed internationally-renowned journals, but not where you'd think to find cutting-edge medical studies. The other reason for this misinformation is that the way we conduct medical studies is not consistent with how integrative and energy-based medical systems work. Integrative and energy-based medicine are very personalized and customized. In other words, we can't study integrative or energy-based techniques by performing the same treatments on a large group of people and observing the results. For example, the treatment of low back pain with acupuncture is very personalized. Different acupuncture points are used in each patient based on the patterns causing the back pain. One client may be diagnosed with a cause of lower back pain called "dampness in the lower jiao with local stasis" whereas another patient may be diagnosed with "liver-kidney deficiency" as a cause of lower back pain. They would receive completely different treatment so we can't use the same acupuncture points in these two clients and expect good results. That's simply NOT how acupuncture works. On the other hand, in conventional allopathic medical studies, the same drug at the same dose would be used to treat all patients in a study with the same diagnosis. If we were studying robots, this method might be effective, but people are not robots and our body function is much too complex to be studied this way. Further, the effectiveness of the drug being studied would be compared to the placebo effect. In conventional medicine, we dismiss the placebo effect as being insignificant, whereas in integrative and energy-based systems of medicine, placebo is critical because we know that our thoughts create chemical reactions in our bodies that determine body function. We become what we think!

The other factor to consider here is that even in conventional allopathic medicine, the standard of care that we practice every day is often *not* based on a large body of scientific evidence. Millions of Americans are on multiple medications and there are no studies done on the effectiveness or potential side effects of taking *multiple* medications together. So, in the case of statins, while we have some idea what a statin alone might do, we have no idea what the combination of a statin with blood pressure medication, diabetes medication, and blood thinners may cause, for example, yet this is done quite frequently. There is no call in the allopathic medical community to conduct medical studies to show that using multiple prescription drugs is safe.

There are many medical and scientific studies to show the efficacy of much of integrative medical practice, but you won't find them in traditional medical journals. Instead you'll find them in *Nature* magazine or *Cell* magazine mostly because we've not yet fostered a culture of true prevention in the United States. Additionally, we haven't yet recognized that medicine is very personalized and therefore not amenable to being studied the way we're used to studying things. In fact, the evidence for integrative medicine can be found in physics research more than in medical research. However, we're well aware of how the human body functions, and if we safely mimic the way the body works and provide the body with the natural ingredients it needs to function, it will. And more importantly, if we provide the energetic support that the body needs, it can heal itself! This is an innate function of the human body. It has a consciousness and an awareness of itself that makes it strive towards efficient function all the time. Even when we're not feeling well, our bodies are working perfectly *with what they have available to them.*

The reason we don't feel well is usually because the body doesn't have the ingredients it needs to function, and/or its path is blocked. Once we know this information, we're can be on our way to promoting wellness.

Ending Our Tolerance of Sickness

Anything less than good health is unacceptable in today's day and age. Wellness should be our default state of being! We have technology today to find out many of the roadblocks to achieving excellent health. TCM gives us a roadmap to follow to regain health and stay well. TCM and functional medicine as practiced in the field of integrative medicine can predict risk of diseases like cancer, Alzheimer's dementia and heart attacks – all valuable information that saves lives once action is taken to correct what's found in order to restore proper body function.

Once we know the body's energy map, we know how to restore good health. If we're depleted, then we know that all our actions should be restorative. We know we should restore ourselves with sleep, rest, breath work, stillness, and light activity. We also know that we should avoid draining activities, such as detoxification and overworking. Over-exercising, such as long-distance running, is also draining and should be avoided when we're depleted. Exercises such as yin yoga, tai chi, and qi gong are more appropriate in this scenario.

If our energy is excessive such as when stagnation or inflammation is present without depletion, we know that we need to do occasional detoxification under the guidance of an expert in this matter. We may benefit from raw vegetable juicing if we're too hot, and we may benefit from spicy broths if we're too cold. This can all be determined by traditional Chinese medicine evaluation. Activities under these circumstances are not as restricted, and consistent movement with exercise is a must. Diet is also critical to avoid introducing more toxins into the body. Household toxins must be more vigilantly eliminated to reduce stagnation or inflammation.

Changing a Mindset, Changing A Culture

Mindset is a popular buzzword today and many researchers are trying to figure out the key to changing mindset and how mindset affects us. Fear-based thinking, which impacts most of us, creates a fixed way of thinking based in survival. It's hard-wired. And it's ubiquitous. It's a hallmark of disease and describes those in category 2 of sickness as we discussed in chapter one. Marketers know based on research that we react more when we're afraid than when we're calm. We're more likely to buy a product based on emotion, especially the emotion of fear. Emotions drive a lot of our behavior, even for the positive things in our lives like our health. We've all been there. We decide we're going to take better care of ourselves and buy a diet book or start an exercise regimen. At first, we're excited and motivated, but after a few days to weeks, our old routines set in and we revert to our usual behaviors. Why? I believe there are two main reasons for this. First, we're more comfortable in our known behaviors than our unknown behaviors. So, if we're not used to eating healthy food options, we're less likely to stick with a new nutrition routine. Our subconscious mind may start thinking about how long it takes to prepare these healthy meals or perhaps how much it costs to purchase them. It also gets bored because it's not getting the usual "fix" from the sugar we're not eating and may set us up to fail. These subconscious thoughts can sabotage us if we're not aware of them and don't prepare for them. We can train ourselves out of this mindset with a little consistent work and mindfulness. In my online program The Wellness Warrior 9-Week Transformation Program, I walk you through the principles of this book and introduce personalized concepts to help you really dig into what's holding you back from experiencing your most vibrant health! Are you struggling with fatigue? Depression? Anxiety? Are you a cancer survivor or perhaps dealing with an ongoing diagnosis of cancer? If so, our community, Awakened Wellness Nation, can help you find the motivation, inspiration and action steps you've been looking for. It'll guide you out of fear and bring you into wholeness to identify the lessons of your illness or symptoms, master self-love, mindfulness and empower you to be and stay well! Learn to navigate through your day, identify what's placing you at risk for disease, choose healthier food options, detox your home and more! There's also an opportunity to ask me questions during our live Q&As as you move through the principles of this book to really lock in the concepts and apply them in your life and your family's life. End the cycle of disease now. The time for a paradigm shift is now!

Learning these concepts for yourself is critical because our culture doesn't reinforce prevention and healthy habits. As we've discussed throughout this book, our allopathic doctor's visit contains almost no discussion of wellness. TV commercials, social media ads, the staples of holiday eating…none of these reinforce wellness or disease prevention. If our culture doesn't inspire and reinforce behaviors that promote wellness, it's extremely difficult to foster lasting changes without consistent support from a reliable source. For more information on our online programs and private community, click here or go to AwakenedWellnessNow.com.

Our culture in America is one of tolerating diseases, but we can change this culture. Research is showing that it doesn't take a majority of people doing something to start an epidemic. Malcolm Gladwell does a great job of explaining this concept in his book, *Tipping Point*. He reviews the research showing that a small percentage of a population can effect massive changes! It's abundantly clear that we shouldn't be waiting for diseases to take hold before taking action. We can and should be more proactive to restore good health and maintain it using the principles of TCM and integrative medicine. Self-empowerment, compassion, and consumer demand will be a critical instrument of change. *Becoming a student of wellness is the only way to wellness. You can't make your own healthcare decisions if you don't know the lay of the land.* Having a poor knowledge of wellness obligates you to follow someone else's lead and disempowers you.

The benefits of traditional Chinese medicine are experiential. They can't be proven in large studies because everyone is a unique individual. The proof comes from that individual feeling well and having that individual's body dysfunction corrected based on proper evaluation and treatment of root causes of symptoms and conditions.

Once proper body function is restored on a cellular and energetic level, we can proceed knowing that our body function is as normal as possible. Our health can be maintained naturally. This requires vigilance and a healthy sense of paranoia to maintain our self-care regimen consisting of mindfulness, stillness, supplements, exercise, and our nutritional regimen every day. *Wellness isn't automatic or passive. It's an active process.* It also requires creating and immersing ourselves in a culture of wellness that reinforces these good habits through support, compassion, and education.

Will we fall off the wagon? Absolutely, but with consistent support and education, we'll get right back on the bandwagon so we know we're moving in the right direction. You can't put a price tag on your health and, just as importantly, you simply can't outspend disease. Latest estimates show that we spend $7,000 per year for each chronic disease we have *despite* insurance coverage. The longer we have a chronic disease, the more expensive it gets over time.

A Thousand-Mile Journey Begins with One Step

Changing the culture of medicine will require an accumulation of people who maintain their health over time using integrative strategies. It'll require consumer demand brought about by a tipping point — a critical number of health-conscious people who are benefiting from this TCM-functional-integrative medical system.

Energy-based science is a fact. It's time we bring it into the realm of medicine, the last frontier to embrace energy-based strategies. Empowering ourselves is the first step in changing the culture of medicine. This generation of children is the first generation in modern times predicted not to live longer than their parents! *The idea that our children can inherit a new system of medicine that's looking into the energy of an individual and seeing the obstacles to body function in order to naturally correct them is the biggest legacy we can leave them.* We're increasingly seeing that natural methods are more effective and safer long-term.

It's time we bring logic into medicine. Requiring evidence for all that we do in medicine isn't logical. The vast majority of medicine as practiced today is not evidence-based and the very nature of how we gather this evidence is flawed. Using the principles we already know about body function and inferring from scientific studies done in other fields such as biology, physics and neurobiology is the best way to proceed while keeping record of outcomes as we move forward while adhering to the principle to do no harm.

Very few medical concepts are proven by scientific study. This is because people are individual, different, and unique. We can't herd them like cattle and do the same treatments and expect them all to be well. That is just not how good health will be brought about in the United States. We need to gauge success one patient at a time. We need to look at patients individually — where they began before assessment and treatment and where they ended based on their individual treatment plans. That's the only successful way to study integrative therapies.

Medical School Education and Integrative Medicine

Educating our frontline physicians to integrate TCM-Functional-Integrative medical guidance strategies and treatments into practice should start in medical school. Experiencing the benefits of this holistic system during a physician's formative years is critical to integrate the system into practice. In 2014, the American Board of Physician Specialties opened the door by accepting the field of integrative medicine as a formal specialty.

Functional medicine principles are easily integrated because they still follow the anatomical principles we're used to. We just have to shift the focus from organs to cells and integrated systems rather than isolated body parts to understand concepts of functional medicine.

Understanding TCM, however, requires emptying our minds and using what are called "beginners' minds" to really absorb and understand TCM's true significance and power. That's what I had to do when I studied it. Continuing to maintain my allopathic medical mind made it almost impossible for me to understand traditional Chinese medicine principles.

TCM-Integrative Medicine As Primary Care

The key to changing the health of Americans for the better requires that TCM-integrative medical systems become a primary point of contact available to a large segment of the population. It shouldn't be a last-minute desperation attempt. Many of my patients come to me after they've exhausted all their other options, and they've been sick for years. Seeking TCM energy-based integrative medical systems early on helps you treat your symptoms much sooner and prevents many diseases. At this time, integrative energy-based principles are usually sought after all other options have been exhausted. This needs to be reversed. We need to flip this principle 180 degrees and accept a new paradigm. An annual ***TCM-Integrative check-up*** should be the first point of contact in order to be effective and applicable to a large segment of the population. It should also be the first point of contact for onset of symptoms that are not life-threatening. For example, if something as simple as a cold is properly treated with clearing herbs or immune-boosting herbs, natural antivirals, or whatever principles are determined to be needed by a TCM-Integrative assessment, then the underlying causes will be treated, and the patient will feel better and preserve their immunity making them healthier overall. How many times have patients experienced being prescribed antibiotics for a cold and ending up on antibiotics over and over again because of recurring symptoms?

These patients need to have their immune systems boosted by appropriate means, not have them torn apart with antibiotics. We need a paradigm shift in order to flip the health of America in the right direction. The American Board of Medical Specialists accepted the field of Integrative Medicine as a medical specialty due to the overwhelming body of evidence showing its usefulness.

Treating minor symptoms early on goes a long way to prevent major conditions that are killing Americans today — Alzheimer's dementia, cancer, heart disease, strokes, and more recently, infections. These are all very preventable if early and minor symptoms such as fatigue, sleep disturbances, frequent colds, etc. are addressed early and successfully by treating their root causes naturally. Making energy-based integrative medical systems a primary point of contact for the majority of Americans will produce a paradigm shift that will be critical to reversing our current course and will help us to successfully transform American medicine into a paradigm of preventing disease and promoting wellness, and not just attempting to prevent death.

The Current Insurance Crisis and Its Solution

Before a system like Integrative medicine can become available to the masses where it's most needed, we must have a system of insurance that allows for the proper use of time for medical visits, empowers physicians and patients to make decisions, and properly reimburses for this work. Currently, our insurance model forces an emphasis on volume of visits rather than quality and complexity. This forces doctors and other health care providers to see as many people as possible in as little time as possible. This is dangerous for professionals because it's not possible to properly focus on wellness in 5-10 minutes, which has increasingly become the average time for a doctor's office visit. Insurance companies also dictate what doctors can do by frequently refusing to pay for medications and procedures prescribed by physicians. Insurance companies are essentially practicing medicine without a license.

A proper integrative wellness visit can take 60-90 minutes for effective results and outcomes. This is because much of integrative medicine focuses on rebuilding the physician-patient relationship, which has been decimated over the past several decades. Patient education and building good habits of self-care are also critical facets of integrative visits. Due to the time-consuming nature of integrative medical care, most integrative medical doctors opt out of insurance and government assistance programs like Medicare.

A solution touted by many medical schools is to provide free medical education for physicians. Their reasoning is that if medical school is free, more doctors will go into allopathic primary care, which is the lowest paying specialty in medicine. In my opinion, even if we flooded the market with allopathic primary care physicians tomorrow, our problems would persist because of the foundational flaws in this allopathic system. The medical system and the way the distribution of funds is currently handled is flawed from top to bottom and requires a drastic overhaul in order to truly reduce the cost of care and inspire wellness in our patients.

Eliminating the 'middle-man' in the insurance paradigm is also critical. One of the unusual things we do in health insurance is cover "maintenance." We cover annual exams and screening tests under health insurance plans. What this does is raise the cost of these assessments because we pay exorbitant premiums for these services and would save much more money if we paid for these services out of pocket. No other insurance model does this. Car insurance doesn't cover car maintenance such as brakes and oil changes. If it did, it would be more costly simply due to the exorbitant administrative costs of managing these simple tasks. Homeowner's insurance doesn't cover maintenance either. If our homeowner's policy covered renovations, painting, home inspections, etc…it, too, would be unaffordable.

The purpose of insurance is to pool risk, not maintenance. Insurance is there in case something goes wrong. Health insurance is the only type of insurance that charges premiums to cover maintenance. It's akin to paying $6.00/gallon for $2.00/gallon's worth of gas! Nobody in their right mind would do this, but we do it every day in health insurance. A better model may be to cover only disease and illness and pay for "maintenance" out of pocket at a market rate which would be considerably lower than what is paid via insurance premiums. This would not only reduce premiums, but combining this with integrative holistic care would slowly reduce the disease burden over time, further reducing healthcare costs long-term. In order to get a system like this off the ground, a fairly healthy younger population would need to participate such as the Millennials, who are the most health-conscious and most willing to spend money on their health, which would make them the ideal generation to kick off a paradigm shift such as this! I don't say this to discriminate against older participants, however, a preventive system cannot work if the majority of the people in that system already have a large burden of disease because you can't prevent what you already have. Older participants who have no current disease burden and are health-conscious would also be ideal candidates.

Keeping funds in the hands of the consumer who is obtaining the integrative care is a critical step in lowering healthcare costs. When we give money to another party such as an insurance broker and ask him to keep what he doesn't spend, nothing good can come of this model except historic profit margins for insurance executives. We've seen this system fail in capitation and in the current insurance model including the affordable care act. Although more people are insured under the ACA, we continue to have unprecedented diseases and healthcare costs. ***We cannot outspend disease***, and until an emphasis on wellness permeates our system it will continue to be unaffordable and risk bankrupting our economy. **A combination of educating and empowering the health care consumer to make his or her own health decisions and having full access to integrative medicine is the long-term key to solving our current healthcare crisis.** Keeping health insurance that covers only illness and accidents would be a safety net as insurance is intended to be. The full solution is well beyond the scope of this book, however, it's imperative to plant the idea that integrative medicine becomes primary care and the payment system shifts to the hands of the consumer and out of the hands of the insurance industry. These are two important principles from which to start. But perhaps the most important of all is to have FAITH: Fearless Affirmation and Intention to Transform Health through the discipline of going within to foster heart-centered living so we can be the best version of ourselves in the world.

"There's courage involved if you want to become truth. There's a broken open place in a lover. Where are those qualities of bravery and sharp compassion in this group? What's the use of old and frozen thought? I want a howling hurt. This is not a treasury where gold is stored; this is for copper. We alchemists look for talent that can heat up and change. Lukewarm won't do. Halfhearted holding back, well-enough getting by? Not here."

-----Rumi as translated by Coleman Barks

In the next chapter, I'll discuss the future of YOU!

CHAPTER NINETEEN

THE FUTURE OF YOU

FAITH: **F**earlessly **A**ffirming and **I**ntending to **T**ransform **H**ealth is a movement towards wellness that starts with you! In reviewing the principles of this book, it's clear that unless each of us makes a conscious choice to look at our health through a different lens, we're virtually guaranteed to get sick and lose the quality of life we've worked so hard to obtain. What does FAITH look like? And where can you begin?

Faith is the belief in something that can't be immediately seen. It's actually more than a belief. It's a knowing…something you don't reason your way to. You just know! Faith is something bigger than we can perceive or believe. Modern science is showing us that there is an alternate reality that we can sense if we look with the right tools. Spooky action at a distance as described by Einstein and proven recently in multiple labs, is giving us a glimpse at this reality that is beyond our universe. Some may call it God or Spirit. Scientists have called it the Field. Either way, it's there and offers us instantaneous communication and contact with something bigger than we are in human form. The Institute of HeartMath® also gives us a glimpse into this other reality through the "heart-brain" which is in instant communication with this other reality! There are scientific studies that show that we can communicate through this reality. Theoretical physicist Nasim Haramein has very elaborate mathematical proofs of the existence of this reality! And ancient traditions have spoken about this other reality for thousands of years!

Communicating with this larger reality creates calm, peace and health that includes resiliency to stress. Why? Stress is a fear-based construct. This larger reality doesn't know fear because it has no meaning there. Communicating with this larger reality allows us to dissolve fear-based thinking and focus on heart-based thinking which brings about feelings of joy, compassion and peace. We become what we think and feel. Feelings of joy and peace lead to wellness. Ancient traditions achieve this through meditation and other practices. Communicating with this larger reality is an experiential practice. It can't be reasoned. The proof is in the experience! That's faith.

Ultimately, the physical body relies on our thoughts to keep it well. Negative thoughts breed disease and positive thoughts breed wellness. Negative thoughts are based in fear. Positive thoughts are based in love. Technically, there are only two emotions: love and fear. We can even suggest that there's only one emotion – love, and that fear is simply the absence or distortion of love. Love and fear can't coexist – we have to ultimately pick one. Believing in love and fear is illogical and is a sign of a split mind. It's a byproduct of duality. As we communicate beyond duality through heart-based thinking and allow the fear to be dissolved, we come to the realization that **there's only love. Everything else is just a cry for help!** Help to do what? Help in transcending fear-based thinking to achieve heart-based thinking and living. How do we know this? We now have scientific evidence that everything is connected. Everything. Numerous studies are showing this. This means that everything we do impacts everyone else on some level. We're all interdependent. Going within ourselves to find peace and love spreads to everyone else. When we see something other than peace and love reflected towards us by others or particular circumstances, it's a sign that we should go further within ourselves to cultivate the positive feelings and thoughts we desire to bring about the wellness of mind and body. This is very empowering because it allows us to be fully in control of our wellbeing. When we're not experiencing fear-based thoughts we can think clearly and steer away from activities or substances that are not life-affirming. This communication with a larger reality steers us to what most benefits us and everyone else.

Ego or fear-based thinking leads to destruction and chaos, as we're increasingly seeing in our world. We've accepted fear as a motivator and its destructive impact can be clearly seen everywhere we look. We can also choose heart-based living and allow this to guide us to wellness. Inspired actions follow from this principle which lead to seeking health models that promote wellness such as traditional Chinese medicine and functional medicine. It can also lead to Ayurveda, yoga, qi gong and any number of other life- and wellness-affirming modalities.

Heart-based thinking and living also inspires us to reduce stress as we begin to see that it's a choice. We can choose to eliminate stress or at least mitigate its impact on our health. Stress isn't an inevitable part of life if we really choose. When we experience and perceive stress, it's a choice to do so whether we recognize it or not. Sometimes the decisions that have to be made to get there feel uncomfortable because they're not choices we're used to making. Sometimes, it's a new job or new relationship, a new home, or a new lifestyle. While it appears to be an impossible road to travel, it's the inevitable conclusion of years of fear-based thinking where we neglected our true needs and health. Heart-based living is the expression of self-love and self-care.

Step #1 on a wellness path is *choosing* heart-based living. How do we begin? Choosing is the first step and committing over and over again on a moment by moment basis is how we stay on the path. Life is not a random event, it's actually an endless series of thoughts. Each thought puts you on a trajectory and your dominant thoughts create your reality. Choose your thoughts wisely! And keep choosing them over and over again. Just deciding once isn't enough. **Life is an endless series of choosing**. *This continuous choosing is called commitment!*

Step #2 on a path to wellness is to learn basic techniques that can reduce stress. In my practice, I teach my clients HeartMath® techniques for coherence. It's important to become a student of the lifestyle you wish to live. I recommend visiting the HeartMath® website for more information as well as practicing the techniques taught there. These techniques are very brief and when consistently practiced, lead to quick and lasting results. Remember, commitment is choosing over and over again to do things that are life-affirming. Doing them a couple times and hoping they stick is like taking 2 baths in your lifetime and expecting to stay clean. It doesn't work. When you commit to life-affirming and heart-based living, the results inspire you to keep moving forward and learn more. Once you've become comfortable with the shorter techniques, you can explore meditation with a teacher or through guided meditations. Not every modality will suit you so be flexible and don't be afraid to try different things until you find what you enjoy doing. Also don't be afraid to move on when you think you've outgrown something. Just be sure that you've found something else which is also life-affirming and heart-based so you don't lose momentum.

Step #3 on a path to wellness includes adequate hydration! 70% of the body by mass is water. 99% of all the molecules in your body are water molecules. That makes water very important. Water is the only known substance to exist in all three phases of matter: gas, liquid and solid. Equally important is the type of water you drink. In order to be safe, water is filtered usually through reverse osmosis. While this takes out dangerous metals and bacteria, it also takes away important minerals. An option may be mineral water as it's sourced from aquifers. According to a study published by the *British Medical Journal*, mineral water can be a good source of calcium, magnesium, bicarbonate, sodium, potassium, and chloride. In general, mineral water sourced from Europe had a more favorable profile. Some mineral waters are acidifying and some are alkalinizing. The higher the sulfate content, the more acidic the water becomes. Alkalinizing mineral waters are generally better and have been shown to be better for bone health among other health benefits. Another caveat is that carbonated mineral waters can thin the enamel on teeth. It's best to vary the brands of mineral waters in order to have a variety of mineral content in your diet. In my private practice, I identify mineral deficiencies in my clients and often recommend that they either re-mineralize their water by adding a small amount of sea salt to their filtered water or taking prescribed minerals. While sea salt is not well studied to date, the preliminary studies are showing it to be superior to processed or refined table salt in terms of mineral content and in health benefits. A study published in 2017 in the journal *Food and Nutrition Research* showed these findings in lab rats. They also showed resistance to high blood pressure in the rats fed sea salt as compared to refined table salt. Hopefully people will be studied soon. Because lab rats and people share similarities, until such studies are performed, we can surmise that adding a small amount of sea salt to our filtered water should be of benefit.

Other great sources of water are spring or mountain water to get EZ-water (exclusion zone water). EZ water is a fourth phase of water made in the body's cells. Regular water has the chemical composition H2O, which is well recognized. EZ water has the chemical composition H3O2 and looks and acts differently inside our cells. When you freeze regular H2O and look under an electron microscope, it doesn't seem to have a structure. However, when you freeze EZ water and look through an electron microscope, this water has the structure of snowflakes and is highly organized! EZ water has specific health benefits as compared to ordinary tap or filtered water. Dr. Masuro Emoto was one of the first to discover this in our modern era. Ancient cultures were well aware of the qualities of spring and mountain water. Multiple studies have now been performed to validate the existence of EZ water. Infrared light causes water to restructure into EZ which means that infrared saunas can restructure the water in your cells even after you drink it! Sunlight is also infrared light especially at dawn and dusk. You can restructure the water in your cells by exposing your core to sunlight at dawn and dusk. Caution should be exercised so that you don't get sunburned or increase your risk of skin cancer. Studies are showing that EZ water helps cells perform their normal functions, improve immunity, and may even kill cancer cells! A study released in the *International Journal of Cell Biology* in 2017 suggested exactly this!

Water temperature. Does it matter? YES! According to TCM, water should be warm and this is highly recommended. Why? The stomach is a hot place. It likes a temperature of approximately 100 degrees. This allows digestive enzymes made by the pancreas to enter the digestive tract and break down the food you eat so that it can be absorbed into the body. Digestive enzymes also allow for proper elimination of waste in the digestive tract. If the stomach is too cold due to consuming cold or iced beverages and foods, digestion and absorption suffers. Given our discussion on the gut (TCM *Spleen*), these properties are critical for good health.

Step #4: Sleep and rest! According to TCM, men require 7 consecutive hours of sleep and women require 8. Why? Remember that women are of blood and men are of qi. Blood is made during sleep making sleep more important for women. If you have a high amount of stress in your life, you'll need even more sleep. If you have adrenal fatigue or feel excessively fatigued in the mornings, more sleep is essential. Another great tip I give my clients is to take afternoon rest. If you can nap, that's best! If you can't nap, take 10-15 minutes between the hours of 1PM-3PM and lay flat with your feet up above your heart to allow the blood to return from the extremities to your core. This is a very refreshing activity that's also great for your health.

Step #5: Eat fresh, organic food sources whenever possible. According to the Environmental Working Group, food is one of the most dangerous sources of toxins that go in our bodies. Many fruits and vegetables are full of pesticides. Sources of protein like poultry, meat and eggs contain artificial ingredients like synthetic hormones, genetically modified grains, antibiotics and more. Grains and dairy are often "fortified" with artificial vitamins, which cause more problems than they solve. Dairy also contains the added toxicity of coming from hormone-fed and GMO-fed cows.

Check a good source such as EWG.org for reports about different foods that are safe to consume. Some tips for finding better food choices include buying only organic fruits and vegetables unless they're on the "Clean 15" list of the EWG. The "Clean 15" has been determined to have a low enough pesticide residue count to be considered safe.

Pasture-raised animals are healthier than caged animals simply because they're less stressed! As we've learned throughout this book, stress makes us unhealthy. Who wants to eat a food source that's not healthy due to stress? Studies show that pasture-raised foods are more nutritious than caged sources. Given what we know about stress, this makes a lot of sense. Read your labels and avoid foods with food coloring and excessive preservatives.

Step #6: Engage in moderate exercise as tolerated. Be sure to have a health screening to assure you're fit enough to exercise. A well-rounded exercise regimen includes strength training as well as endurance training. Consult with a health coach or trainer to get you off to a good start. Intense exercise isn't always best. Listen to your body when you exercise and remember it's talking to you at all times! If you feel exhausted immediately after or the next day, you've done too much and should rest and do less next time. Find that sweet spot and increase your endurance gradually so it's tolerable and not too stressful. Don't forget to be outdoors to get fresh air and to engage with nature. Just being in a natural environment is healing!

Step #7: Declutter your life of unnecessary activities that aren't restorative. For example, many Americans stay up watching TV or playing video games to wind down from their day. While this may provide some immediate gratification, it doesn't serve to restore you. You may consider sitting quietly outside in nature and doing a deep breathing exercise, walking, or reading a good book. Doing some gratitude work by writing a short paragraph in a journal about what happened that day for which you're grateful is also a very restorative activity. The 6 Healing Sounds of Taoism is a great way to restore. As mentioned earlier, you can read about this in Mantak Chia's book *Chi Nei Tang*. And, of course, HeartMath® training with the Quick Coherence Technique is a phenomenally restorative activity and it only takes 3 minutes!

Step #8: Remove dangerous toxins from your home. Many people are unaware of the numerous toxins that surround them in their own home. Most people are exposed to 200 cancer-causing toxins almost daily. These same toxins capable of causing cancer can also increase the risk of other diseases like autism, autoimmune diseases, and more. The Environmental Working Group has done great work in this area. Visit EWG.org for more information. They also have an app you can download onto your phone to make it easier to shop.

Removing toxins from the home is a time-consuming step so remember that slow and steady wins the race. It's difficult to rid your home of all toxins, so perfection isn't the goal here. The more you can remove, the less the toxic burden on your body. Household cleaning products, makeup, lotions, and foods are the big categories. The easiest way to clear your home is to look at what's about to run out and look up cleaner and greener alternatives before you run out. Then you can pick up the healthier alternative instead of buying the toxic one again. While this option may seem expensive when you do a price comparison, it's critical to realize that investing in better health is always the more cost-effective route to take. Disease is always a losing investment! While organic strawberries may cost more than regular strawberries, the avoidance of cancer or gastrointestinal disorders this toxic food can cause is worth its weight in gold! When we add up co-pays and deductibles for doctors' visits and the intangible cost of not feeling good, being less productive at work, or not being able to participate in the activities you love with your family and friends, spending more on healthier options becomes easier. Don't forget about your air conditioning filters. Make sure you get HEPA filters and change them as recommended to remove circulating toxins from your home.

Step #9: Protect yourself from electromagnetic frequency (EMF) and radio frequency (RF) pollution. Electromagnetic radiation and radio frequency pollution is becoming a public health hazard. Sources of radio frequency include microwaves, cell phones, televisions, smart meters, and computers. In May 2011, the International Agency for Research on Cancer classified radio frequency as category 2B: a possible human carcinogen. Additional studies since that time have strengthened the association between RF pollution and cancer; however, most countries have not taken significant action to protect their citizens, so that leaves it up to you! A particularly strong association has been made between cell phones and brain tumors. The device used to detect and measure EMF/RF exposure in a study conducted by the *International Journal of Oncology* was the EME Spy 200 by MVG. A more cost-effective option is the Trifield meter. For more information about EMF/RF, I recommend the book *Zapped* by Ann Louise Gittleman. A strategy to minimize your exposure is to make sure you don't have a television, computer or cell phone in your bedroom. Devices to reduce or absorb the frequencies are also available. The only way to know if the devices to reduce EMF/RF exposure work is to measure both before and after applying them to your devices, home or person. The meter should reflect a reduction to accepted levels if the device is working appropriately. There are currently no reliable guidelines regarding safe levels of exposure so less is best until we can get more data. Given that we know that our bodies are energy fields that are powered by electricity, it's easier to see how electromagnetic and radio waves that aren't in alignment with our bodies can damage them. Antioxidant-rich foods are a great source to reduce the impact of EMF/RF exposure. A study published in *Nutrition Journal* in 2010 measured the antioxidant levels of over 3,100 foods. Certain categories of foods and beverages made the list of highest anti-oxidant levels. Foods such as herbs and spices like allspice, turmeric, and cloves had the highest anti-oxidant levels. Berries high in anti-oxidants are Indian gooseberry, bilberries, wild strawberries, black currants, blackberries, and cranberries. Espresso also qualifies as a high anti-oxidant beverage and bested green tea! Dark chocolate with high cocoa content also made the list. Shelled nuts have higher anti-oxidant value than nuts already out of the shell. Keeping the pellicles on certain seeds and nuts preserves their antioxidant content. Pellicles are the thin layer, membrane, or skin around a seed or nut. Walnuts, pecans, sunflowers and chestnuts had the highest anti-oxidant levels in the nuts/seeds category. Again, nature has built-in protective mechanisms to keep us healthy so why not take advantage of them!

Step #10: Invest in your wellness by seeing a board-certified integrative medical doctor who has certification in Chinese medicine or another form of energy-based medicine to take advantage of the fact that we are electromagnetic energy beings and not just physical bodies.

To learn how to put these recommendations and the information in this book to work for your wellness, go to AwakenedWellnessNow.com where you'll find our online programs and our private community Awakened Wellness Nation that help you navigate through these recommendations and help the words on the pages come to life for you. In this supportive space, you'll find like-minded individuals ready to share their stories, insights, and experiences. Together, we'll explore topics that matter to you, from personal growth and mindset shifts to holistic health practices and self-care strategies. Join us for engaging discussions, interactive workshops, and valuable resources designed to inspire you to take charge of your health and wellbeing. Whether you're seeking motivation, accountability, or simply a space to connect, our online community, Awakened Wellness Nation, is your sanctuary for growth and empowerment. Let's embark on this transformative journey together and awaken the best version of ourselves. I'm dedicated to making this brand of medicine accessible to as many people as possible. The future of YOU is very bright if you have FAITH: Fearless Affirmation and Intention to Transform Health! I hope I've inspired you to join me on the path to prevention and wellness. It'll take a movement which starts with each of us to create consumer demand that will force a paradigm shift around the globe to change our sick-care model to the healthcare model it should be.

You don't have to be a statistic - your life, your children, your loved ones, and the entire world depend on you not becoming one. I wish you many blessings on your journey and thank you for your open mind and heart.

WORKS CITED

Arregger, AL, LN Contreras, OR Tumilasc, DR Aquilano, and EM Cardoso. "Salivary Testosterone: A Reliable Approach to the Diagnosis of Male Hypogonadism." Clinical Endocrinology (Oxford). 2007 Nov:67(5):656-62.

Ashley Winning, M. Maria Glymour, Marie C. McCormick, Paola Gilsanz and Laura D. Kubzansky; Psychological Distress Across the Life Course and Cardiometabolic Risk Findings From the 1958 British Birth Cohort Study; Journal of the American College of Cardiology; Volume 66, Issue 14, October 2015; DOI: 10.1016/j.jacc.2015.08.021

Badwe, RA, DY Wang, WM Gregory, IS Fentiman, MA Chaudary, P. Smith, MA Richards, and RD Rubens. "Serum Progesterone At the Time of Surgery and Survival in Women with Premenopausal Operable Breast Cancer." European Journal of Cancer. 1994:30A(4):445-8.

Bancel, P., Nelson, R., The GCP Event Experiment: Design, Analytical Methods, Results. Journal of Scientific Exploration, 2008. 22(3): p. 309-333.

Beach, Rex. "Modern Miracle Men. U.S. Senate Document 264. Presented by Mr. Fletcher 5 Jun 1986.

Bernstein, L., JM Yuan, RK Ross, MC Pike, R. Hanisch, R. Lobo, F. Stanczyk, YT Gao, and BE Henderson. "Serum Hormone Levels in Pre-Menopausal Chinese Women in Shanghai and White Women in Los Angeles: Results from Two Breast Cancer Case-Control Studies." Cancer Causes Control. 1990 Jul:1(1):51-8.

Bertolote, JM, A. Fleischmann, M. Eddleston, and D. Gunnell. "Deaths from Pesticide Poisoning: Are We Lacking A Global Response?" British Journal of Psychiatry. Author manuscript 2006 Sep:189: 201–203. doi: 10.1192/bjp.bp.105.020834, PMCID: PMC2493385, EMSID: KMS1629.

Bog-Hieu Lee, Ae-Ri Yang, Mi Young Kim, Sara McCurdy, William A. Boisvert; Natural sea salt consumption confers protection against hypertension and kidney damage in Dahl salt-sensitive rats; Food Nutr Res. 2017; 61(1): 1264713. Published online 2016 Dec 20. doi: 10.1080/16546628.2017.1264713

Brauser, Deborah. "Probiotics: A Potential Treatment for Mental Illness." Medscape MedicalNews,Psychiatry.Nov19,2013. http://www.medscape.com/viewarticle/814672. 2016.

Campagnoli, Carlo, Francoise Clavel-Chapelon, Rodolf Kaaks, Clementina Peris, and Franco Berrino. "Progestins and Progesterone in Hormone Replacement Therapy and the Risk of Breast Cancer." Journal of Steroid Biochemistry and Molecular Biology 96 (2005) 95-108.

Canonico, M., E. Oger, G. Plu-Bureau, J. Conard, G. Meyer, H. Lévesque, N. Trillot, MT Barrellier, D. Wahl, J. Emmerich, and PY Scarabin. "Hormone Therapy and Venous Thromboembolism Among Postmenopausal Women: Impact of the Route of Estrogen Administration and Progestogens: the ESTHER Study." Estrogen and Thromboembolism Risk (ESTHER) Study Group. Circulation. 2007 Feb 20:115(7):840-5.

Cardoso, EM, AL Arregger, OR Tumilasci, and LN Contreras. "Diagnostic Value of Salivary Cortisol in Cushing's Syndrome (CS)." Clinical Endocrinology (Oxford). 2009 Apr:70(4):516-21. doi: 10.1111/j.1365-2265.2008.03381.x. Epub 2008 Aug 15.

Chang, KJ, TT Lee, G. Linares-Cruz, S. Fournier, and B. de Lignieres. "Influences of Percutaneous Administration of Estradiol and Progesterone on Human Breast Epithelial Cell Cycle in Vivo." Fertility and Sterility. 1995 Apr:63(4):785-91.

Chang, C. J., Lin, C. S., Lu, C. C., Martel, J., Ko, Y. F., Ojcius, D. M., et al. (2015). Ganoderma lucidum reduces obesity in mice by modulating the composition of the gut microbiota. *Nat. Commun.* 6, 7489. doi: 10.1038/ncomms8489

Chatterjee, Anusuya, Sindhu Kubendran, Jaque King, and Ross DeVol. "Check-Up Time: Chronic Disease and Wellness in America. Measuring the Economic Burden in A Changing Nation." Milken Institute Review. Jan 2014.

Christina D. Bethell PhD, MBA, MPH , Michael D. Kogan PhD, Bonnie B. Strickland PhD, Edward L. Schor MD, Julie Robertson, Paul W. Newacheck DrPH "A National and State Profile of Leading Health Problems and Health Care Quality for US Children: Key Insurance Disparities and Across-State Variations" Academic Pediatrics Volume 11, Issue 3, Supplement, May–June 2011, Pages S22-S33

Cowan, LD, L. Gordis, JA Tonascia, and GS Jones. "Breast Cancer Incidence in Women with A History of Progesterone Deficiency." American Journal of Epidemiology. 1981 Aug:114(2):209-17.

Crimmins, EM, SH Preston, B. Cohen, eds. United States, National Research Council Panel on Understanding Divergent Trends in Longevity in High-Income Countries. "Explaining Divergent Levels of Longevity in High-Income Countries." Washington, DC. National Academies Press (US), 2011.

Davani-Davari D, Negahdaripour M, Karimzadeh I, et al. Prebiotics: Definition, Types, Sources, Mechanisms, and Clinical Applications. *Foods*. 2019;8(3):92. Published 2019 Mar 9. doi:10.3390/foods8030092

DeVol, Ross and Armen Bedroussian. "An Unhealthy America: The Economic Burden of Chronic Disease. Charting a New Course to Save Lives and Increase Productivity and Economic Growth." Milken Institute Review. Oct 2007.

Everhart, JE, ed. "The Burden of Digestive Diseases in the United States." Bethesda, MD: National Institute of Diabetes and Digestive and Kidney Diseases, U.S. Department of Health and Human Services; 2008. NIH Publication 09–6433.

Fairweather, DeLisa and Noel R. Rose. "Women and Autoimmune Diseases 1." Emerging Infectious Diseases Nov 10.11 (2004):2005–11. doi: 10.3201/eid1011.040367. PMCID: PMC3328995. 2016.

Fournier, Agnes, Franco Berrino, Elio Riboli, Valerie Avenel, and Francoise Clavel-Chapelon. "Breast Cancer Risk in Relation to Different Types of Hormone Replacement Therapy in E3N-EPIC Cohort." International Journal of Cancer. Apr 10: 114(3):448-54 (2005).

Fournier, et al. "Unequal Risks for Breast Cancer Associated with Different Hormone Replacement Therapies: Results from the E3N Cohort Study." Breast Cancer Research and Treatment. 2008 Jan:107(1):103-11.

Fournier, et al. "Use of Different Postmenopausal Hormone Therapies and Risk of Histology- and Hormone Receptor-Defined Invasive Breast Cancer." Journal of Clinical Oncology. 2008 Mar 10:26(8):1260-8.

Fowler AA 3rd, Truwit JD, Hite RD, et al. Effect of Vitamin C Infusion on Organ Failure and Biomarkers of Inflammation and Vascular Injury in Patients With Sepsis and Severe Acute Respiratory Failure: The CITRIS-ALI Randomized Clinical Trial [published correction appears in JAMA. 2020 Jan 28;323(4):379]. JAMA. 2019;322(13):1261-1270. doi:10.1001/jama.2019.11825

Geschwind DH. Genetics of autism spectrum disorders. *Trends Cogn Sci.* 2011;15(9):409-416. doi:10.1016/j.tics.2011.07.003

Goodman, Professor Alissa (principal investigator). "1958 National Child Development Study." Centre for Longitudinal Studies.

Gozansky, WS, JS Lynn, ML Laudenslager, and WM Kohrt. "Salivary Cortisol Determined by Enzyme Immunoassay Is Preferable to Serum Total Cortisol for Assessment of Dynamic Hypothalamic-Pituitary-Adrenal Axis Activity." Clinical Endocrinology (Oxford). 2005 Sep:63(3):336-41.

Herrera AY, Nielsen SE, Mather M. Stress-induced increases in progesterone and cortisol in naturally cycling women. Neurobiol Stress. 2016;3:96–104. Published 2016 Feb 11. doi:10.1016/j.ynstr.2016.02.006

Hollingsworth, Dr.P.H., Carol M. Ashton, M.D., M.P.H., and Nelda P. Wray, M.D., M.P.H. "A Controlled Trial of Arthroscopic Surgery for Osteoarthritis of the Knee." New England Journal of Medicine 2002:347:81-88 July 11, 2002. DOI: 10.1056/NEJMoa 013259.

Huang TL[1], Charyton C. A comprehensive review of the psychological effects of brainwave entrainment. Alternative Therapies in Health and Medicine, 2008 Sep-Oct;14(5):38-50.

Hwang SG, Hong JK, Sharma A, Pollack GH, Bahng G. Exclusion zone and heterogeneous water structure at ambient temperature. *PLoS One*. 2018;13(4):e0195057. Published 2018 Apr 18. doi:10.1371/journal.pone.0195057

Janicki, Sarah C., MD, MPH and Nicole Schupf, PHD, DrPH. "Hormonal Influences on Cognition and Risk for Alzheimer Disease." Current Neurology and Neuroscience Report. Author Manuscript 2010 Sep:10(5): 359–366. doi: 10.1007/s11910-010-0122-6. PMCID:PMC3058507. NIHMSID: NIHMS271579.

Kang DH, Lim HW, Lee WY, Jee YS (2018) Faster Recuperation of Pain and Musculoskeletal System through Vibroacoustic Sound Therapy. Journal of Biology and Medical Research Vol.2 No.1:5

"Killer Environment." Environmental Health Perspectives. Feb 107.2 (1999): A62-3.

Kirsh, V. and N. Kreiger. "Estrogen and Estrogen-Progestin Replacement Therapy and Risk of Post-Menopausal Breast Cancer in Canada." Cancer Causes Control. 2002 Aug:13(6):583-90.

Klein, Eric A., MD; Ian M. Thompson, MD; Catherine M. Tangen, DrPH; John J. Crowley, PhD; M. Scott Lucia, MD; Phyllis J. Goodman, MS; Lori M. Minasian, MD; Leslie G. Ford, MD; Howard L. Parnes, MD; J. Michael Gaziano, MD, MPH; Daniel D. Karp, MD; Michael M. Lieber, MD; Philip J. Walther, MD, PhD; Laurence Klotz, MD; J. Kellogg Parsons, MD, MHS; Joseph L. Chin, MD; Amy K. Darke, MS; Scott M. Lippman, MD; Gary E. Goodman, MD; Frank L. Meyskens, MD; Laurence H. Baker, DO. "Vitamin E and the Risk of Prostate Cancer: The Selenium and Vitamin E Cancer Prevention Trial." Journal of the American Medical Association. 2011: 306(14):1549-1556. doi:10.1001/jama.2011.1437.

Klein, I. and S. Danzi. "Thyroid Hormone Treatment to Mend A Broken Heart." The Journal of Clinical Endocrinology & Metabolism. 2008 Apr: 93(4): 1172–1174.

Kowalski K, Mulak A. Brain-Gut-Microbiota Axis in Alzheimer's Disease. J Neurogastroenterol Motil. 2019;25(1):48-60. doi:10.5056/jnm18087

Langley, RL and SA Mort. "Human Exposures To Pesticides in the United States." Journal of Agromedicine. 2012:17(3):300-15. doi: 10. 1080/1059924X.2012.688467.

L'Hermite, et al. "Could Transdermal Estradiol +Progesterone Be A Safer Postmenopausal HRT? A Review." Maturitas 2008:60(3), 185-201.

Lili Naghdi MD CCFP,1,2 Heidi Ahonen, PhD MTA,1,3 Pasqualino Macario, DC,2 and Lee Bartel, PhD; The effect of low-frequency sound stimulation on patients with fibromyalgia: A clinical study. Pain Research and Management 2015 Jan-Feb; 20(1): e21–e27

Liu, Sha, Honghai Wu, Gai Xue, Xin Ma, Jie Wu, Yabin Qin, and Yanning Hou, MD. "Metabolic Alteration of Neuroactive Steroids and Protective Effect of Progesterone in Alzehimer's Disease-Like Rats." Neural Regeneration Research. 2013 Oct 25:8(30): 2800–2810. doi:10.3969/j.issn.1673-5374.2013.30.002. PMCID: PMC4146013.

Luciana Terra, Paul J. Dyson, Matthew D. Hitchings, Liam Thomas, Alyaa Abdelhameed, Ibrahim M. Banat, Salvatore A. Gazze, Dušica Vujaklija, Paul D. Facey, Lewis W. Francis, Gerry A. Quinn. A Novel Alkaliphilic Streptomyces Inhibits ESKAPE Pathogens. Frontiers in Microbiology, 2018; 9 DOI: 10.3389/fmicb.2018.02458

McKay, LA, TR Holford, and MB Bracken. "Re-Analysis of the PREGNANT Trial Confirms That Vaginal Progesterone Reduces the Rate of Preterm Birth in Women with a Sonographic Short Cervix." Ultrasound in Obstetrics & Gynecology. 2014 May:43(5):596-7. doi: 10.1002/uog.13331. Epub 2014 Apr 7.

Magnusson, C., JA Baron, N. Correia, R. Bergström, H. Adami, and I. Persson. "Breast-Cancer Risk Following Long-Term Oestrogen-and Oestrogen-Progestin-Replacement Therapy." International Journal of Cancer. 1999 May 5:81(3):339-44.

Manish Arora, Abraham Reichenberg, Charlotte Willfors, Christine Austin, Chris Gennings, Steve Berggren, Paul Lichtenstein, Henrik Anckarsäter, Kristiina Tammimies, Sven Bölte. Fetal and postnatal metal dysregulation in autism. Nature Communications, 2017; 8: 15493 DOI: 10.1038/NCOMMS15493

Marais A et al. 2018 The future of quantum biology. J. R. Soc. Interface 15: 20180640. http://dx.doi.org/10.1098/rsif.2018.0640

McCraty, R., M. Atkinson, and R.T. Bradley, Electrophysiological evidence of intuition: Part 1. The surprising role of the heart. Journal of Alternative and Complementary Medicine, 2004. 10(1): p. 133-143.

McCraty, R., M. Atkinson, and R.T. Bradley, Electrophysiological evidence of intuition: Part 2. A system-wide process? Journal of Alternative and Complementary Medicine, 2004. 10(2): p. 325-336

McCraty, R., Barrios-Choplin, B., Rozman, D. et al. The impact of a new emotional self-management program on stress, emotions, heart rate variability, DHEA and cortisol; Integrative Physiological and Behavioral Science (1998) 33: 151. https://doi.org/10.1007/BF02688660

McMaster University, Hamilton, ON, Canada; Brain-Body Institute, St. Joseph's Healthcare, Hamilton, ON, Canada.

Meltzer, A., Van de Water, J. The Role of the Immune System in Autism Spectrum Disorder. *Neuropsychopharmacol* **42,** 284–298 (2017). https://doi.org/10.1038/npp.2016.158

Mohr, PE, DY Wang, WM Gregory, MA Richards, and IS Fentiman. "Serum Progesterone and Prognosis in Operable Breast Cancer." British Journal of Cancer. 1996 Jun:73(12):1552-5.

Monica H Carlsen, Bente L Halvorsen, Kari Holte, Siv K Bøhn, Steinar Dragland, Laura Sampson, Carol Willey, Haruki Senoo, Yuko Umezono, Chiho Sanada, Ingrid Barikmo, Nega Berhe, Walter C Willett, Katherine M Phillips, David R Jacobs, Jr, Rune Blomhoff.

Moseley, J. Bruce, M.D., Kimberly O'Malley, Ph.D., Nancy J. Petersen, Ph.D., Terri J. Menke, Ph.D., Baruch A. Brody, Ph.D., David H. Kuykendall, Ph.D., John C. The total antioxidant content of more than 3100 foods, beverages, spices, herbs and supplements used worldwide; *Nutr J.* 2010; 9: 3. Published online 2010 Jan 22. doi: 10.1186/1475-2891-9-3

Moskowitz A, Andersen LW, Huang DT, et al. Ascorbic acid, corticosteroids, and thiamine in sepsis: a review of the biologic rationale and the present state of clinical evaluation. Crit Care. 2018;22(1):283. Published 2018 Oct 29. doi:10.1186/s13054-018-2217-4

Naik, Shruti et al. Two to Tango: Dialog between Immunity and Stem Cells in Health and Disease. Cell, Volume 175, Issue 4, 908 – 920
Nataliya Petryk, Maria Dalby, Alice Wenger, Caroline B. Stromme, Anne Strandsby, Robin Andersson, Anja Groth. MCM2 promotes symmetric inheritance of modified histones during DNA replication. Science, 2018; eaau0294 DOI: 10.1126/science.aau0294

National Institutes of Health, U.S. Department of Health and Human Services. "Opportunities and Challenges in Digestive Diseases Research: Recommendations of the National Commission on Digestive Diseases." Bethesda, MD: National Institutes of Health; 2009. NIH Publication 08–6514.

Nelson, R., Effects of Globally Shared Attention and Emotion. Journal of Cosmology, 2011. 14.

Nowakowski, Matilda E., Randi McCabe, Karen Rowa, Joe Pellizzari, Michael Surette, Paul Moayyedi, and Rebecca Anglin. "The Gut Microbiome: Potential Innovations for the Understanding and Treatment of Psychopathology." Canadian Psychology/Psychologie Canadienne, Vol 57(2), May 2016:67-75. http://dx.doi.org/10.1037/cap0000038.

O'Leary, P., P. Feddema, K. Chan, M. Taranto, M. Smith, and S. Evans. "Salivary, but Not Serum or Urinary Levels of Progesterone Are Elevated After Topical Application of Progesterone Cream to Pre- and Postmenopausal Women." Clinical Endocrinology (Oxford). 2000 Nov:53(5):615-20.

Otsuki, M., H. Saito, X. Xu, et al. "Progesterone, But Not Medroxyprogesterone, Inhibits Vascular Cell Adhesion Molecule-1 expression in Human Vascular

Endothelial Cells." Arteriosclerosis, Thrombosis, and Vascular Biology. 2001 Feb:21(2):243-8.

Qu Z., Cui J., Harata-Lee Y., Aung T., Feng Q., Raison J. M., Kortschak R., Adelson D. L. Identification of candidate anti-cancer molecular mechanisms of Compound Kushen Injection using functional genomics. Oncotarget. 2016; 7: 66003-66019. Retrieved from https://www.oncotarget.com/article/11788/text/

Romero, Roberto, M.D. "Vaginal Progesterone to Reduce the Rate of Preterm Birth and Neonatal Morbidity: A Solution At Last." HHS Author Manuscripts. Women's Health (London, England). Author manuscript. 2011 Sep:7(5): 501–504. doi: 10.2217/whe.11.60.

Romero, R., L. Yeo, P. Chaemsaithong, T. Chaiworapongsa, and SS Hassan. "Progesterone to Prevent Spontaneous Preterm Birth." Seminars in Fetal and Neonatal Medicine. 2014 Feb:19(1):15-26. doi:10. 1016/j.siny.2013.10.004. Epub 2013 Dec 5.

Rosano, GM, CM Webb, S. Chierchia, et al. "Natural Progesterone, But Not Medroxyprogesterone Acetate, Enhances the Beneficial Effect of Estrogen on Exercise-Induced Myocardial Ischemia in Post-menopausal Women." Journal of the American College of Cardiology. 2000 Dec:36(7):2154-9.

Sarne D. Effects of the Environment, Chemicals and Drugs on Thyroid Function. [Updated 2016 Sep 27]. In: Feingold KR, Anawalt B, Boyce A, et al., editors. Endotext [Internet]. South Dartmouth (MA): MDText.com, Inc.;2000. https://www.ncbi.nlm.nih.gov/books/NBK285560/

Spencer, CP, IF Godsland, AJ Cooper, D. Ross, MI Whitehead, and JC Stevenson. "Effects of Oral and Transdermal 17Beta-Estradio with Cyclical Oral Norethindrone Acetate on Insulin Sensitivity, Secretion, and Elimination in Postmenopausal Women." Metabolism. 2000 Jun:49(6):742-7.

Strydom, C, C. Robinson, E. Pretorius, JM Whitcutt, J. Marx, and MS Bornman. "The Effect of Selected Metals on the Central Metabolic Pathways in Biology: A Review." Department of Anatomy, School of Health Sciences, Faculty of Health Sciences, University of Pretoria, PO Box 2034, Pretoria, 0001, South Africa.

Highveld Biological Association, Sandringham, Johannesburg, South Africa, Departments of Urology, School of Medicine, Faculty of Health Sciences, University of Pretoria, South Africa. Water SA Vol.32 (4) 2006: pp.543-554.

United Nations. "Chemical Risk: The Muted Crisis. A Few Steps in the Right Direction at the ICCM3. ICCM 3. Nairobi, 2014.

U.S. Centers for Disease Control and Prevention. Second National Report on Biochemical Indicators of Diet and Nutrition in the U.S. Population 2012. Atlanta (GA): National Center for Environmental Health; April 2012.

USGS: ca.water.usgs.gov/pnsp/atmos/atmos_1.html.

Van Vugt, Marieke Karlijn, Peter Hitchcock, Ben Shahar, and Willoughby Britton. "The Effects of Mindfulness-Based Cognitive Therapy on Affective Memory Recall Dynamics in Depression: A Mechanistic Model of Rumination." Frontiers in Human Neuroscience 19 Sep 2012. http://dx.doi.o10.3389/fnhum.2012.00257. 2016.

Waheed, S., Kafaei, J. (2018). 'A review on Medication Heavy Metals and Current Assay Methods', *Medbiotech Journal*, 02(04), pp. 136-141. doi: 10.22034/mbt.2018.80816

Winning, A., MM Glymour, MC McCormick, P. Gilsanz, and LD Kubzansky. "Psychological Distress Across the Life Course and Cardiometabolic Risk: Findings from the 1958 British Birth Cohort Study." Journal of the American College of Cardiology. 2015:66(14):1577-1586. doi:10.1016/j.jacc.2015.08.021.

World Health Organization, radiofrequency radiation and health - a hard nut to crack (Review); Lennart Hardell; Int J Oncol. 2017 Aug; 51(2): 405–413. Published online 2017 Jun 21. doi: 10.3892/ijo.2017.4046

World Health Organization. (2015). Serum and red blood cell folate concentrations for assessing folate status in populations. World Health Organization. https://apps.who.int/iris/handle/10665/162114

Writing Group for the Women's Health Initiative Investigators. "Risks and Benefits of Estrogen Plus Progestin in Healthy Postmenopausal Women: Principal Results from the Women's Health Initiative Randomized Controlled Trial. Journal of the American Medical Association. 2002:288(3):321-333. doi:10.1001/jama.288.3.321.

Wynn, E., Raetz, E., & Burckhardt, P. (2008). The composition of mineral waters sources from Europe and North America in respect to bone health: Composition of mineral water optimal for bone. British Journal of Nutrition 101 (8), 1195-1199. Doi: 10.1017/S0007114508061515

Xu, J., Lian, F., Zhao, L., Zhao, Y., Chen, X., Zhang, X., et al. (2013). Structural modulation of gut microbiota during alleviation of type 2 diabetes with a Chinese herbal formula. 9, 552–562. doi: 10.1038/ismej.2014.177

Yan Shao, et al., Stunted microbiota and opportunistic pathogen colonization in caesarean-section birth, September 2019; Nature; https://doi.org/10.1038/s41586-019-1560-1

Yan Zhang, Yanxue Xue, Shiqiu Meng, Yixiao Luo, Jie Liang, Jiali Li, Sizhi Ai, Chengyu Sun, Haowei Shen, Weili Zhu, Ping Wu, Lin Lu, Jie Shi. Inhibition of Lactate Transport Erases Drug Memory and Prevents Drug Relapse. Biological Psychiatry, 2016; 79 (11): 928 DOI: 10.1016/j.biopsych.2015.07.007

Yang, Y., Chen, G., Yang, Q., Ye, J., Cai, X., Tsering, P., et al. (2017). Gut microbiota drives the attenuation of dextran sulphate sodium-induced colitis by Huangqin decoction. *Oncotarget* 8, 48863–48874. doi: 10.18632/oncotarget.16458

Yegambaram M, Manivannan B, Beach TG, Halden RU. Role of environmental contaminants in the etiology of Alzheimer's disease: a review. *Curr Alzheimer Res.* 2015;12(2):116-146. doi:10.2174/1567205012666150204121719

Zhang Y, Han M, Liu Z, Wang J, He Q, Liu J. Chinese herbal formula xiao yao san for treatment of depression: a systematic review of randomized controlled trials. *Evid Based Complement Alternat Med.* 2012;2012:931636. doi:10.1155/2012/931636

Zhou L, Foster JA. Psychobiotics and the gut-brain axis: in the pursuit of happiness. Neuropsychiatr Dis Treat. 2015 Mar 16;11:715-23. doi: 10.2147/NDT.S61997. PMID: 25834446; PMCID: PMC4370913.

INDEX

www.ingramcontent.com/pod-product-compliance
Lightning Source LLC
Chambersburg PA
CBHW021543260326
41914CB00001B/136

* 9 7 8 0 5 7 8 7 9 1 2 7 2 *